12 LEAD EKG STAT!
A LIGHT-HEARTED APPROACH
Second Edition

Donna Memoly Koenig RN, BA, CCRN
Staff Nurse CCU
St. Peters Medical Center, New Brunswick, New Jersey
Instructor
School of Cardiovascular Technology
Morristown Memorial Hospital, Morristown, New Jersey

Denise Topp RN, ADN, CCRN
Staff Nurse CCU
St. Peters Medical Center, New Brunswick, New Jersey

Laura Gasparis Vonfrolio RN, MA, CEN, CCRN
Staff Development Instructor
St. Vincent's Medical Center, Staten Island, New York
Assistant Professor of Nursing
College of Staten Island, Staten Island, New York
President
Education Enterprises & A.D. Von Publishers,
Staten Island, New York

CEU Access Books
Parsippany, New Jersey

CEU Access Books
20 Camelot Road
Parsippany, New Jersey 07054

Cartoons by Donna Memoly Koenig

12 LEAD EKG STAT!

A LIGHT-HEARTED APPROACH

Second Edition

ISBN 0-9631206-0-3

© 1992 by CEU Access. Copyright under the Uniform Copyright Convention. All rights reserved. This book is protected by copyright. No part of it may be reproduced, stored in a retrieval system or transmitted in any form or by any means, electronic, mechanical, photocopying, recording or otherwise, without written permission from the publisher. Made in the United States of America. Library of Congress catalog card number 92-70155

Last digit is the print number: 9 8 7 6 5 4 3 2 1

Printed on Recycled Paper ∞

DEDICATED TO:

Raymond J. Memoly

Frank S. Pack

James Gasparis

SPECIAL THANKS TO:

Ashok Kumar M.D., F.A.C.C., F.A.C.P.
Clinical Associate Professor
Robert Wood Johnson University Hospital
New Brunswick, New Jersey

Robert M. Pickoff M.D.

ACKNOWLEDGEMENTS

Janet Bonanno
Linda Bosworth
Cecilia Claye
Christopher Delaney
Lina Doyle
Carolyn Fleischmann
Fay Gasparis
Annette Jarrett
Melinda L. Lambert
Barbara J. Memoly
Mark S. Memoly
Rosie Miller
Gregorio Rue
Araceli U. Ruiz
Donald Topp
Arlene R. Vitanza
Charles Vonfrolio
Kathleen Wagner
Robert L. Wang
Peter White
St. Peters Medical Center CICU Staff

LETTER TO OUR READERS:

Dear Colleague,

We're so excited that you are the proud owner of a new innovative approach to 12 Lead EKG Interpretation, called **12 Lead EKG STAT!** *A Light-Hearted Approach. EKG's have been made to be a complex topic, a mind-boggling tedious journey. Hey! Kick your shoes off as this adventure is made to be fun! Don't be surprised if at times you find you're not in Kansas anymore, but in EKG fairytale land, reading about Prince Ischemia and Princess Infarction. You will even have energy left over at the end of the book to complete a test for CEU's and work a 12 hour shift!*

In the back of the book, there are two answer forms for the CEU test. Photocopies are acceptable. Share the book with your friends so that they too may earn CEU's. Happy Reading!

DMK
DT
LGV

Table of Contents

SECTION ONE
WITHIN NORMAL LIMITS
An EKG Fairytale Begins 2
Leads - A Point of View 7
Electrical Conduction 23
Complexes and Intervals 30
The "Normal" EKG 44
Axis Deviation 54

SECTION TWO
MYOCARDIAL INFARCTION
The Fairytale Continues 62
The Coronary Arteries 68
Landscape of Myocardial Infarction 74
Infarction, Wall to Wall 84
Pericarditis 98

SECTION THREE
HYPERTROPHY, BUNDLE BRANCH BLOCK, AND ECTOPY
The Fairytale Continues 104
Chamber Enlargement and Hypertrophy 108
Bundle Branch Blocks 118
Hemiblocks 135
Aberration versus Ectopy 141

SECTION FOUR
Appendix: Depolarization 151
The Fairytale Concludes 152
Bibliography 166
Index 167
CEU Test 175
Answer Sheets and Evaluation Forms 193

SECTION ONE

WITHIN NORMAL LIMITS

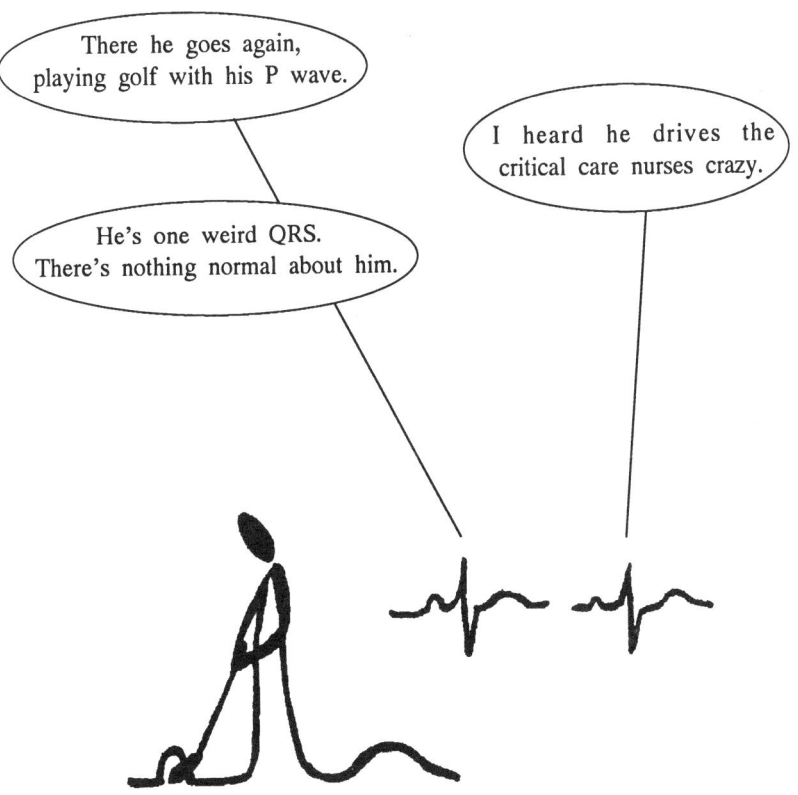

The Little Princess with a Q Wave

An EKG Fairytale Begins . . .

Royal Hypochondria

"*I'm sure there's something wrong with me — do the EKG again — please.*" The youngest prince of the Royal House of Cholesterol plucked the lemon linen fabric of his designer suit for a few moments, he thought, **all this Doctor ever worries about is my sister!** He said, "*Isn't it true that an EKG can look perfectly normal even when there's a real and serious problem underneath? Isn't it true that a patient's story is the most important thing?*"

The prince was in his cardiologist's office so often that Dr. Finebeat had dubbed him Prince Ischemia. Occasionally he would see inverted T waves in the inferior leads of his EKGs and sometimes there was some ST depression also. All the cardiac medications he prescribed for him were ignored, however, so the doctor was frustrated and a little mystified as to what Prince Ischemia wanted from him.

"*Yes, that is true. In fact—*" began nurse Zephanie Z. Zucker, reflecting back on an EKG book she had just read ... something with a light-hearted approach ...

Dr. Finebeat silenced her with a single post-cards-from-the-edge glance, said, "*We've done thirty seven EKGs on you this month. Your five cardiac caths this year showed clean* arteries, we could not induce spasms." His voice lost its cool even tone at the end of that pathetic observation. His mother would have called it whining. Sunlight streaming through the venitian blinds caught highlights in his glorious black hair as the doctor shook his head, no more EKGs today.

"Maybe we could do a set of cardiac enzymes," suggested Nurse Zucker.

Dr. Finebeat wanted to throw himself around the room but he managed magnificent self-control. It was one of the things nurses liked most about him. He knew he was very popular with them. Anyway Zephanie was new to his office, sharp and observant, so he wouldn't let himself get upset that she was encouraging this crazy royal in his obsession.

"Bloodwork?" inquired the prince hopefully.

"We usually like to keep the enzymes and other lab work down to once a month, right prince? said the doctor.

"Oh, I didn't realize —" said the nurse.

"Here, go for it," Dr Finebeat said, handing Zephanie a syringe.

The prince watched carefully as Zephanie drew the blood and placed it in a test tube with a red stopper. As soon as the tube was labelled with his name, the prince clutched his chest and screamed, "Oh, the pain — midsternal, constant, throbbing, radiating to my arm, my jaw, my ... foot."

"How about a right-sided EKG?" said Stephanie.

"What's a right-sided EKG?" asked Prince Ischemia, suddenly calm.

Why me, wondered Robert Finebeat. **Why was I**

appointed to this position? He said, "His majesty has no signs of a right-sided infarct. He's not hypotensive, there's no jugular venous distention, his heart tones are clear."

"I can't believe you never mentioned this right-sided EKG to me before," snarled the prince.

Dr. Finebeat felt his temples begin to throb. "We have done a number of right-sided EKGs on you," he said. "Remember when there was a line of leads on the right side of your chest?"

"Well, what's the difference? What does it mean," snapped Prince Ischemia.

"Think of it as just a different point of view," said Zephanie. "All those little leads are like eyeballs looking into your heart."

"I command that you do a right-sided EKG this minute," said Prince Ischemia the Great. "I need all the eyeballs I can get."

WITHIN NORMAL LIMITS

COGNITIVE OBJECTIVES

* Identify the bipolar and unipolar leads
* Name and identify the position of the precordial leads.
* Identify placement of the leads in a right-sided EKG.
* Describe the MCL_1 lead.
* Describe the hexaxial reference system.
* Describe the portion of the heart muscle viewed by each lead.
* Describe the pathway of electrical conduction in a healthy heart.
* Identify the shapes and times of normal complexes and intervals.
* Identify right and left axis deviation in a 12 lead EKG.

LEADS - A POINT OF VIEW

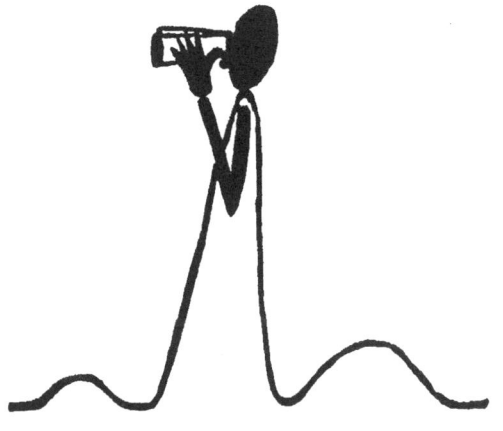

LEADS, A POINT OF VIEW

A lead is a view of the electrical activity of the heart which can be traced in sweeping arcs of excitement across the skin. There are bipolar leads and unipolar leads.

A *bipolar* lead is composed of one positive and one negative electrode. A *unipolar* lead is composed of a positive electrode and a neutral reference point that is determined by the EKG machine. The neutral reference point lies close to the heart. The positive electrode of any lead is considered the seeing eye of the lead.

The direct path between two electrodes or between one electrode and a reference point is called the *axis* of the lead. The tracing of activity registered by the EKG machine *is the lead.* Try to think of a lead as a recording of the electrical activity between two points.

Axis of the Lead

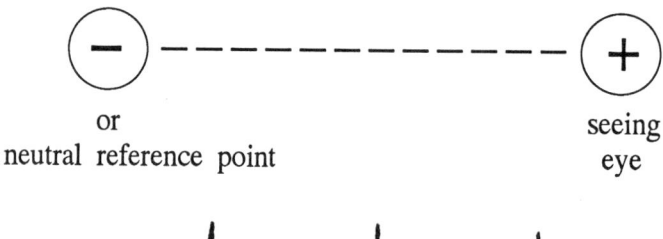

or
neutral reference point

seeing
eye

A lead is a tracing of activity

Not surprisingly there are twelve leads in a 12-lead EKG. Three of these leads are bipolar: leads I, II and III. Nine of the leads are unipolar: aVR, aVL, aVF, V_1, V_2, V_3, V_4, V_5, and V_6. All these leads examine the walls of the heart. We have more leads than walls, thus there is overlapping of the views of the heart.

BIPOLAR LEADS

Lead I: Lead I has a positive electrode on the left arm and a negative electrode on the right arm. It views the lateral wall. When in Lead I the EKG machine makes the right arm negative and the left arm positive.

Lead I: Lateral Wall

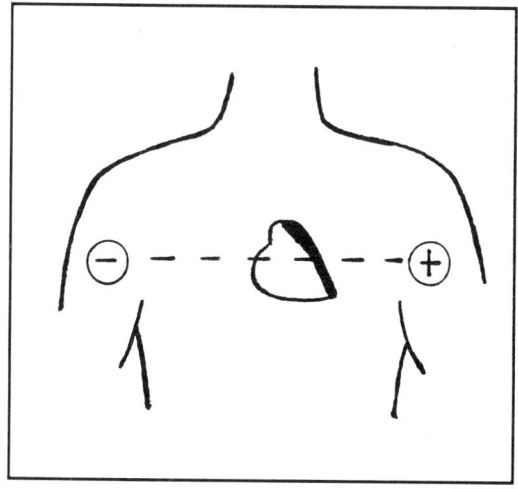

Lead II: Lead II *moves the positive electrode* to the left leg while the negative electrode remains on the right arm. Lead II glances up across the chest from left to right and watches the inferior wall. When in Lead II the EKG machine makes the electrode on the left leg positive and keeps the right arm negative.

Lead II: Inferior Wall

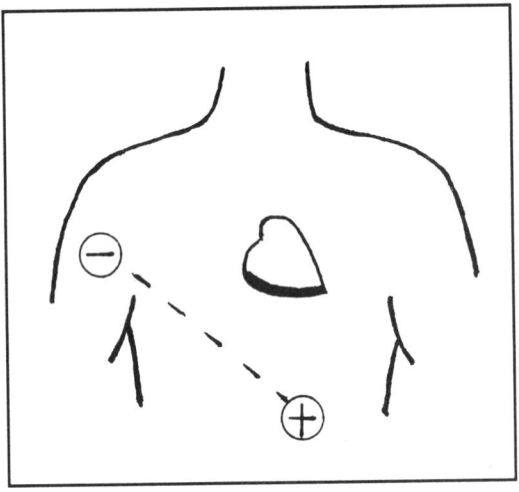

Lead III: The positive electrode remains on the left leg while the negative electrode moves to the left arm. The left leg continues to peer up over the heart but its gaze changes direction. Lead III is a different portrayal of the inferior wall. When in Lead III, the machine keeps the left leg positive and makes the left arm the negative point.

Lead III: Inferior Wall

UNIPOLAR LEADS

Remember — in a unipolar lead there is a positive electrode and a neutral reference point. The neutral reference point is determined by averaging the electrical potentials of other leads. There are unipolar *limb* leads and unipolar *chest* leads

Unipolar Limb Leads

aVR: This lead is the only one that views events from way out in right field, so to speak. Some people call this the orphan lead because normally no electrical current from the heart comes its way. The "a" in aVR stands for "augmented." Unipolar limb leads need a little boost of current to make their appearances readable. (When Einhoven invented the EKG machine, he made sure the recording of aVR, aVL and aVF was 50% bigger so you can see it.)

aVR: ? Orphan Lead

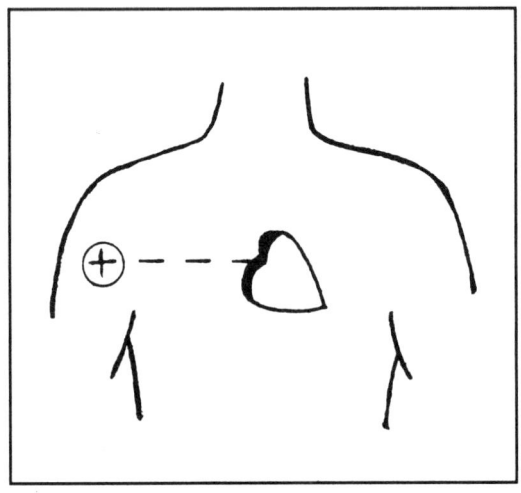

12

aVL: aVL has a positive electrode that sits on the left arm and a neutral reference point close to the heart. aVL inspects the lateral wall.

aVL: Lateral Wall

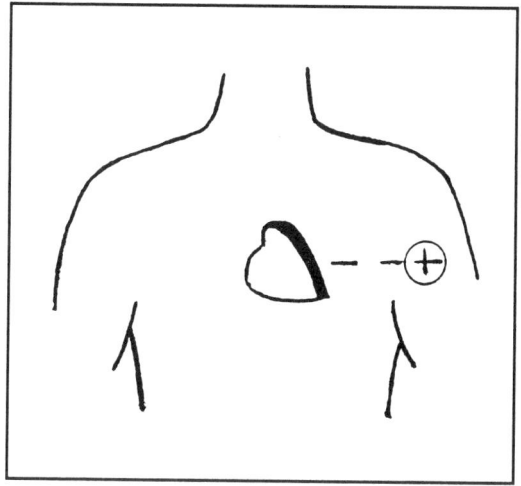

aVF: aVF keeps in touch with the heart from the left foot. It's another inferior wall lead. If it studies the inferior wall, it is a limb lead. You could say aVF is just another limb-lead inferior-wall watcher.

aVF: Inferior Wall

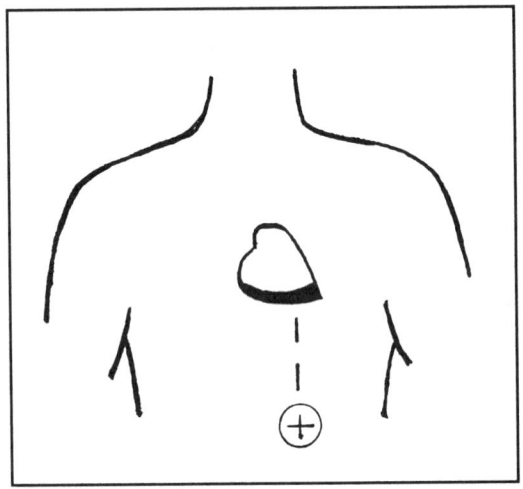

Unipolar and bipolar limb leads — leads I, II, III, aVR, aVL, and AVF are also known as *frontal* leads.

Chest or Precordial Leads

It makes sense that a cluster of leads around the heart would yield a wealth of information. The precordial or "V" leads are unipolar leads encircled around the precordium and do just that.

Leads V_1 through V_4 view the anterior wall while leads V_1 and V_2 delineate activity of the ventricular septum as well. V_5 and V_6 examine the lateral wall. Chest leads have their axes in a horizontal plane because they are so near to the heart.

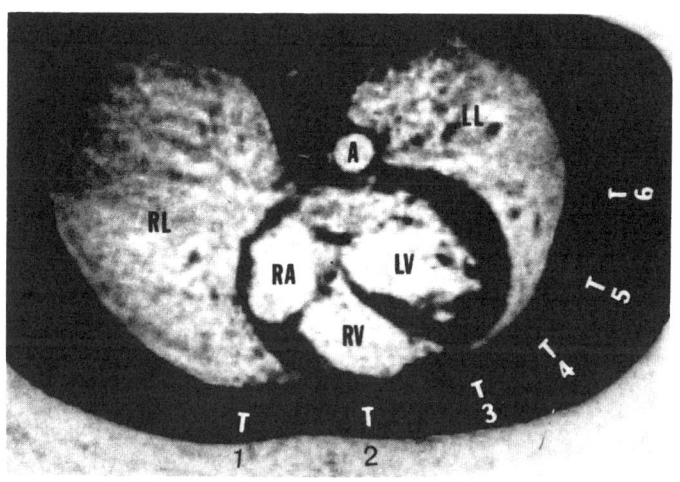

Magnetic resonance image of heart to illustrate approximate relationship of chest electrodes to cardiac chambers. Points 1-6 represent sites of the six precordial electrodes. V_1-V_6, RA = right atrium; RV = right ventricle; LV = left ventricle; RL = right lung; LL = left lung; A = aorta. *Reprinted with the permission of W.B. Saunders in Philadelphia and the author. From <u>Practical Electrocardiography</u>, 1988, 8th Edition, by Henry J.L. Marriott, M.D., F.A.C.P., F.A.C.C.*

V_1 — V_4: Anterior Wall
V_1 — V_2: Ventricular Septum
V_5 — V_6: Lateral Wall

Placement of Precordial Leads

V_1: 4th intercostal space at right sternal border
V_2: 4th intercostal space at left sternal border
V_3: Midway between V_2 and V_4
V_4: 5th intercostal space at left midclavicular line
V_5: 5th intercostal space at left anterior axillary line
V_6: 5th intercostal space at left midaxillary line

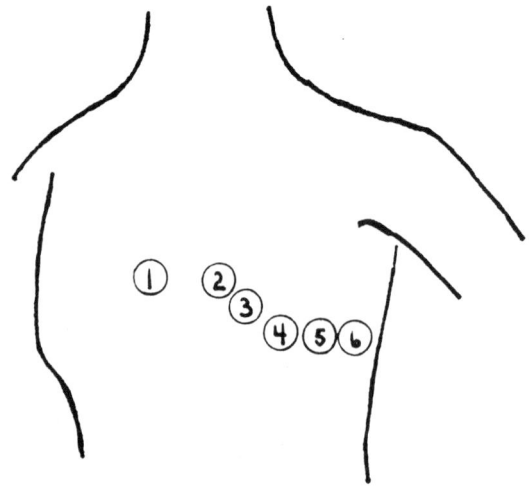

ADDITIONAL LEADS

Sometimes you find your patient complaining of severe chest pain and the 12-lead EKG shows slight changes or none at all. You might want to try some different leads.

Right-Sided EKGs

Right-sided lead placement mirrors a standard EKG but the leads are placed on the right side of the chest. This is used when the patient has an inferior wall infarction, as the right ventricle gets damaged along with the left ventricle 30% of the time. It is also useful when a patient shows clinical signs of right-sided infarction such as hypotension with jugular venous distension.

Right-Sided Placement

V_1R: 4th intercostal space at left sternal border

V_2R: 4th intercostal space at *right* sternal border

V_3R: Midway between V_2R and V_4R

V_4R: 5th intercostal space at *right* midclavicular line

V_5R: 5th intercostal space at *right* anterior axillary line

V_6R: 5th intercostal space at *right* midaxillary line

RIGHT-SIDED EKG

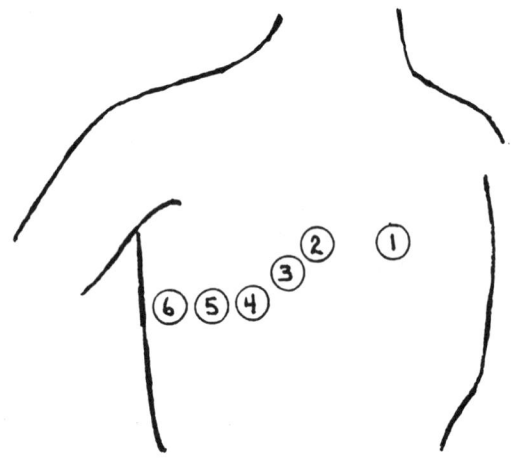

Marvelous MCL₁
For Constant Monitoring

When you are monitoring a rhythm continuously, as in a telemetry or critical care setting, you should use MCL_1. MCL_1 is a modified chest lead that mimics V_1. It gives a lot of information regarding the interpretation of bundle branch blocks. It is also useful in the differential diagnosis of ventricular ectopy versus aberrantly conducted beats.

If you see ectopy on the monitor, call for a twelve-lead EKG. Look at more than one lead. In the meantime, keep your patient in MCL_1 because if you have only one little strip to look at and the ectopy has vanished by the time you get into the patient's room – then this is the best view you'll get.

MCL_1

Right 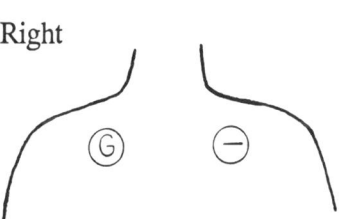 Left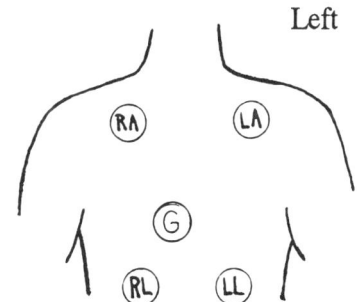

On a 3-lead system—put the monitor in lead 1. Place the left arm (+) electrode at the 4th intercoastal space at the right sternal border and the right arm (-) electrode on the left shoulder.

On a 5-lead system—Put the monitor in MCL_1. Place the electrodes where they normally go but be sure to put the ground at the 4th intercoastal space at the right sternal border.

AN EKG RIDDLE

What is kind of crazy, seems to make no sense, and used widely by experts in the field?
The hexaxial reference system.

The Hexaxial Reference System

Hexaxial reference is a system in which all *frontal* leads lie in precise relation to one another. First picture leads I, II, and III forming a triangle. This famous figure is known as Einthoven's triangle. The next step is to move these leads toward each other until they intersect.

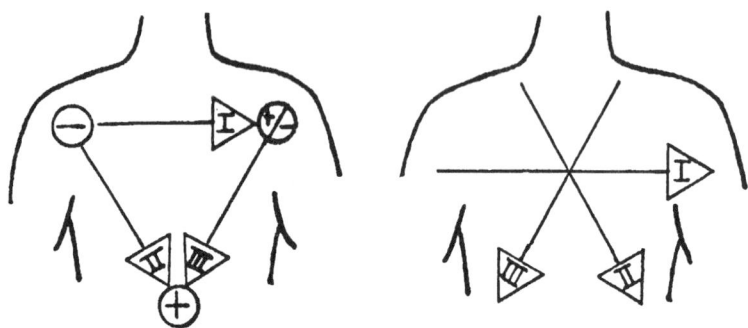

Einthoven's
Triangle

Note that while the intersected leads maintain *parallel directions,* leads II and III seem to have traded places.

Next . . .

Hexaxial Reference

Next Leads aVR, aVL, and aVF are added.

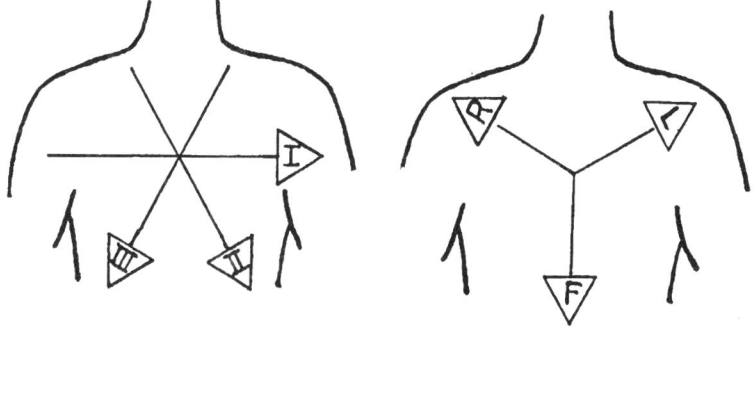

Voila:

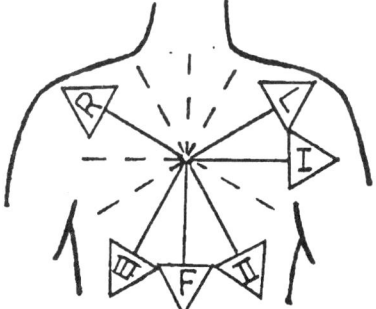

Hexaxial reference is used for landmarks in the following **Roadmap to the Leads.**

ROADMAP TO THE LEADS

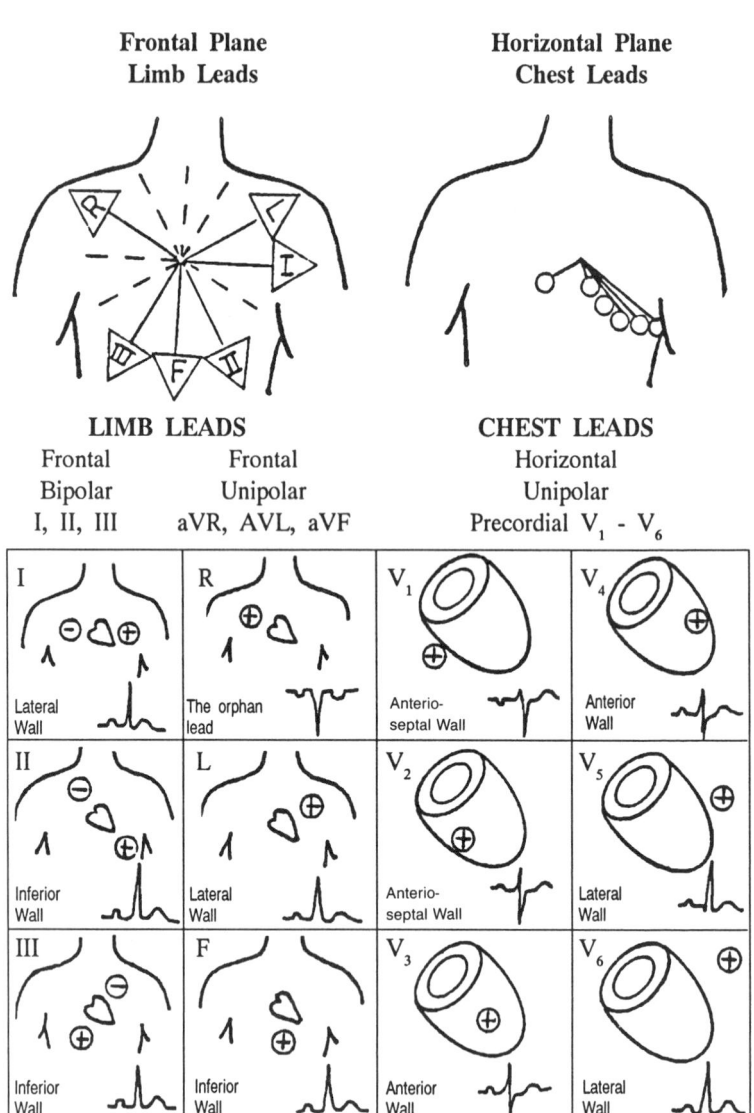

ELECTRICAL CONDUCTION

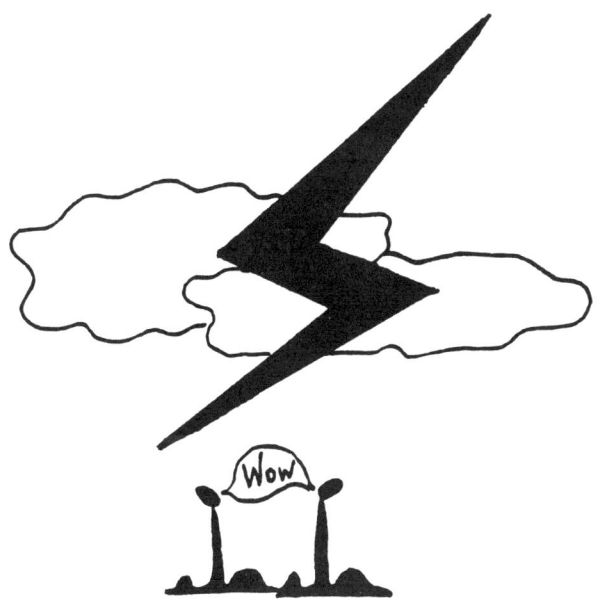

YOUR ELECTRIC HEART

A thick mass of special cells that depolarize automatically and faster than any other cells begin each heartbeat with a burst of electrical energy. These cells make up the *sinoatrial (SA) node*. A resultant wave of excitation sweeps through potassium and sodium, calcium and magnesium ions, making muscle ready to move. The SA node is located in the *right* atrial wall below the superior vena cava.

The electrical impulse journeys across to the left atrium via an interatrial pathway called *Bachmann's Bundle* and down to the *atrioventricular (AV) node* through internodal pathways. The AV node is also in the right atrium but it is near the bottom of the atrial septum and is one of the last places in the atrial to depolarize.*

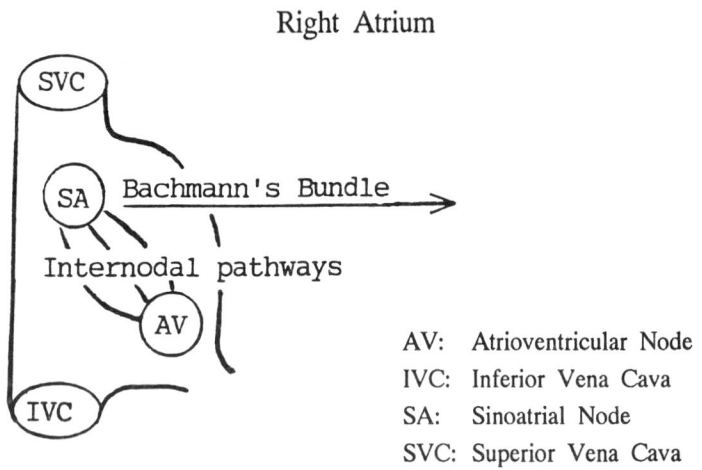

AV: Atrioventricular Node
IVC: Inferior Vena Cava
SA: Sinoatrial Node
SVC: Superior Vena Cava

* For a description of depolarization, see Appendix.

At the AV node, conduction slows to a near crawl due to the nature of the conduction cells there. This allows time for blood to fill the ventricles. When the AV node is fully depolarized, the atria contract and we see a P wave on the EKG.

 a P wave

This wave of energy trekking through the heart has magnitude (size) and direction and so it qualifies as a *vector*.

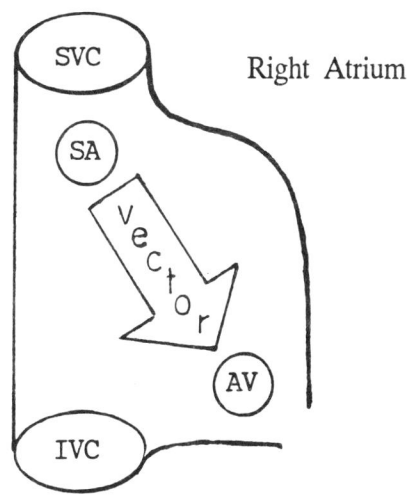

A vector is a quantity possessing magnitude and direction.

When the vector of cardiac excitation emerges from the AV node, it picks up speed and races into the bundle of HIS and onto the bundle branches.

The left bundle branch sends tiny divisions of itself to electrify the ventricular septum before it splits into two major fascicles: the anterior-superior fascicle and the posterior-inferior fascicle. The *left* bundle branch depolarizes *before* the right bundle branch; the impulse travels across the septum.

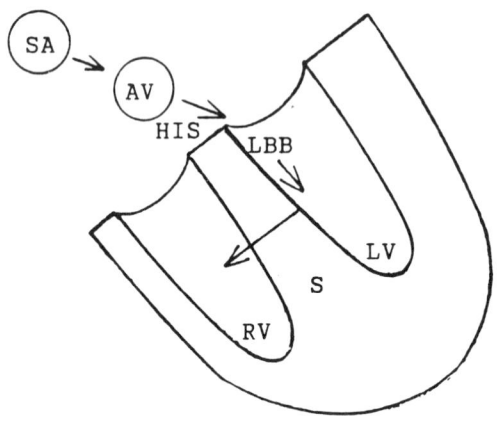

SA:	Sinoatrial Node	LBB:	Left Bundle Branch
AV:	Atrioventricular Node	RV:	Right Ventricle
HIS:	Bundle of HIS	LV:	Left Ventricle
S:	Septum		

From the bundle branches the vector streams into a diffuse network of Purkinje fibers which coat the endocardium of both ventricles. Conduction time through Purkinje fibers is very fast.

As the impulse travels through the AV node, the Bundle of HIS, the bundle branches and the Purkinje fibers, we see a P-R interval (PRI) on the EKG. When the Purkinje fibers depolarize, the ventricles contract simultaneously and a QRS appears.

P wave: Atrial contraction

PRI: Depolarization of
       AV node
       Bundle of HIS
       Bundle Branches
       Purkinje Fibers

QRS: Ventricular
       contraction

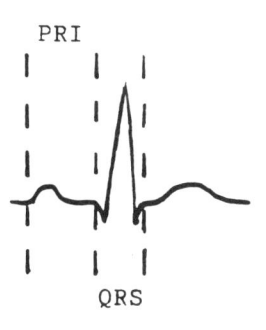

During ventricular systole the atria relax. We don't see this relaxation on an EKG because it is swallowed by the strong QRS complex. When the ventricles relax (or repolarize) a T wave appears. Occasionally a U wave follows a T wave. The significance of U waves has not been established. They may represent recovery of the Purkinje fibers or papillary muscles. They appear more readily in the presence of electrolyte imbalance, certain drugs and left ventricular hypertrophy.

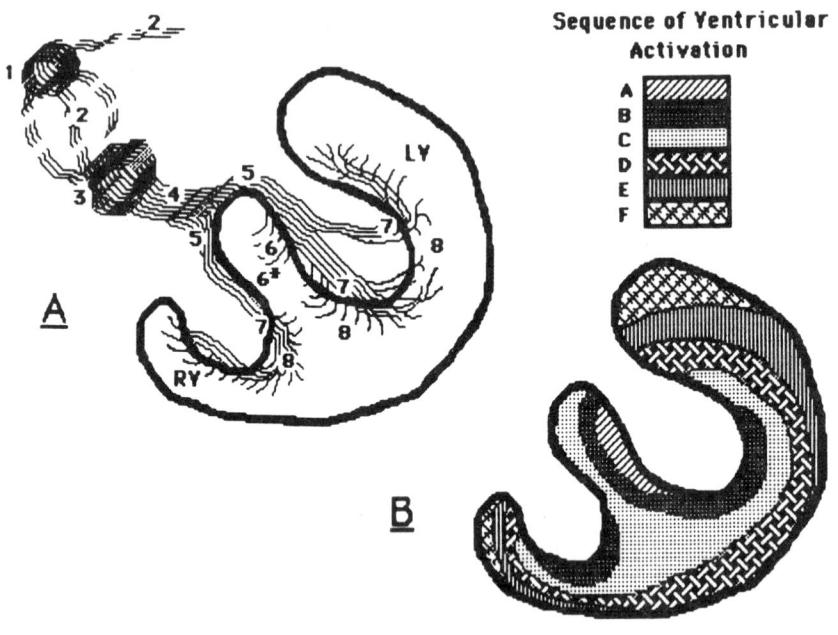

A. Atrioventricular conduction system. B. Sequence of ventricular activation. LV - Left ventricle; RV - Right Ventricle; 1 - SA node: 2 - Interatrial and internodal tracts; 3 - AV node; 4 - Bundle of His; 5 - Division of His into left and right bundle branches; 6 - First activation of the septum of arborizations from the left bundle branch; 6 - Spread of electrocial impulse through the septum 7 - Travel through distal bundle branch system; 8 - Exit from terminal ramifications of Purkinje system. *Reprinted from Clinical Electrocardiography: A Primary Care Approach by Ken Grauer, M.D. and R. Whitney Curry Jr., M.D. A Medical Economics Book reprinted with permission of Blackwell Scientific Publications in Cambridge, MA. 1987*

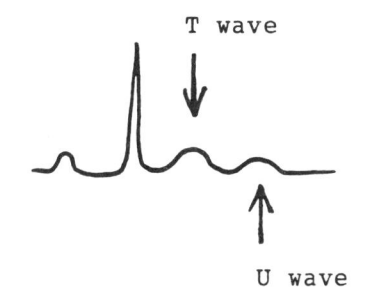

T Wave: Repolarization of ventricles

U Wave: Recovery of Purkinje Fibers or Papillary muscles?

At any given moment in the cardiac cycle, we can measure and plot the various surges of energy happening to determine an "instantaneous vector." More useful is the *net or mean cardiac vector* which portrays the summation of the waves of excitation, their direction and size, from beginning to end of the cardiac cycle.

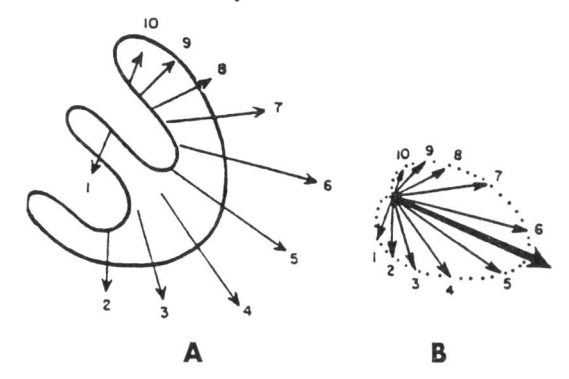

(A) Diagram of successive instantaneous axes (or vectors) as the ventricular muscle mass is depolarized. (B) Regrouping of the instantaneous vectors in as though they all originated from a single "center"; the thick arrow represents the *mean* vector, being the resultant of the 10 instantaneous vectors. *Adapted from* Practical Electrocardiography *by Henry J.L. Marriott, M.D., F.A.C.P., F.A.C.C. Reprinted with permission of the publisher, Williams and Wilkins in Baltimore and with permission of the author.*

In a healthy heart the mean cardiac vector travels downward from right to left. This is the normal axis of the electrical circuit of the heart.

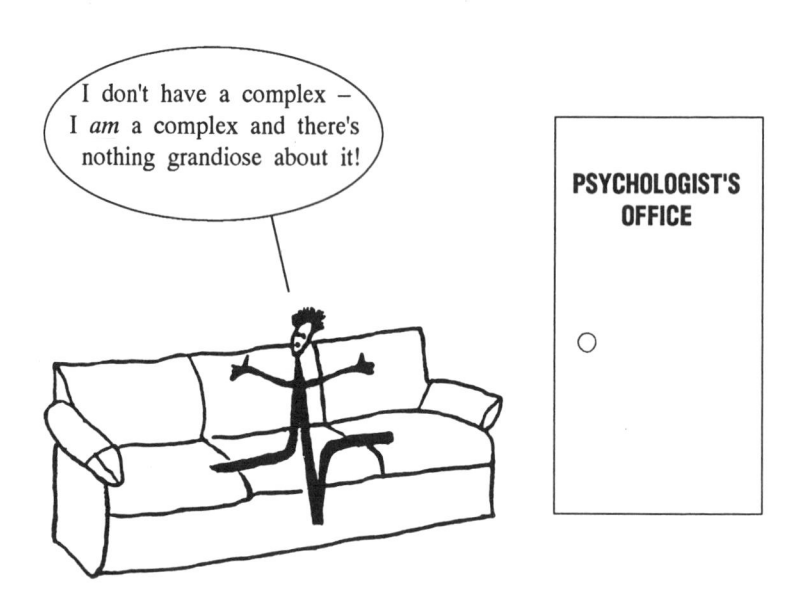

COMPLEXES AND INTERVALS

I don't have a complex — I am *a complex and there's nothing grandiose about it!*

PSYCHOLOGIST'S OFFICE

SHAPES AND TIMES OF COMPLEXES AND INTERVALS

EKG paper is scored horizontally and vertically. There are big boxes and baby boxes. A baby box is one square millimeter. Along a horizontal axis (EKG people love the word, axis) a baby box signifies 0.04 seconds. A big box is comprised of five baby boxes. Along a horizontal axis a big box signifies 0.20 seconds.

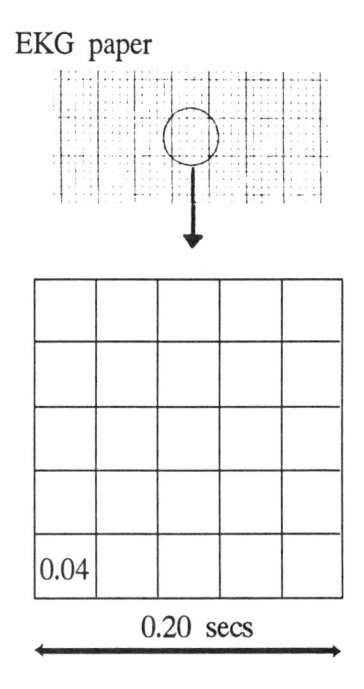

EKG paper

0.04

0.20 secs

Along a vertical axis, one baby box represents 0.1 millivolt while a big box represents 0.5 millivolt. EKG complexes and intervals are drawn against this stark but exact background.

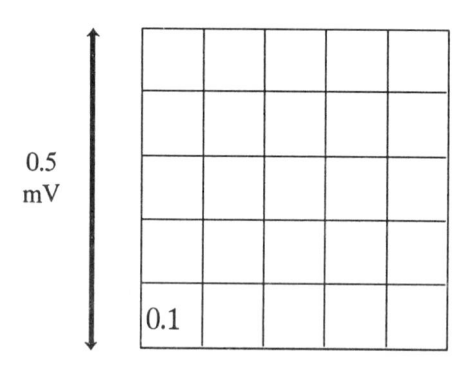

P WAVES

The P wave depicts atrial depolarization. Normally it does not exceed 0.11 seconds and has a rounded shape. A peaked P wave indicates enlargement of the right atrium (P-pulmonale) while notching of the P wave indicates enlargement of the left atrium (P-mitrale).

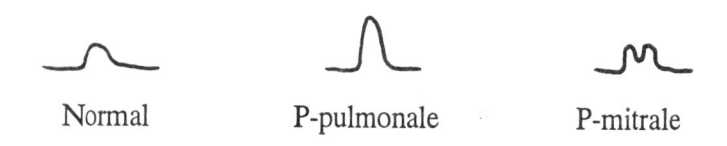

Normal   P-pulmonale   P-mitrale

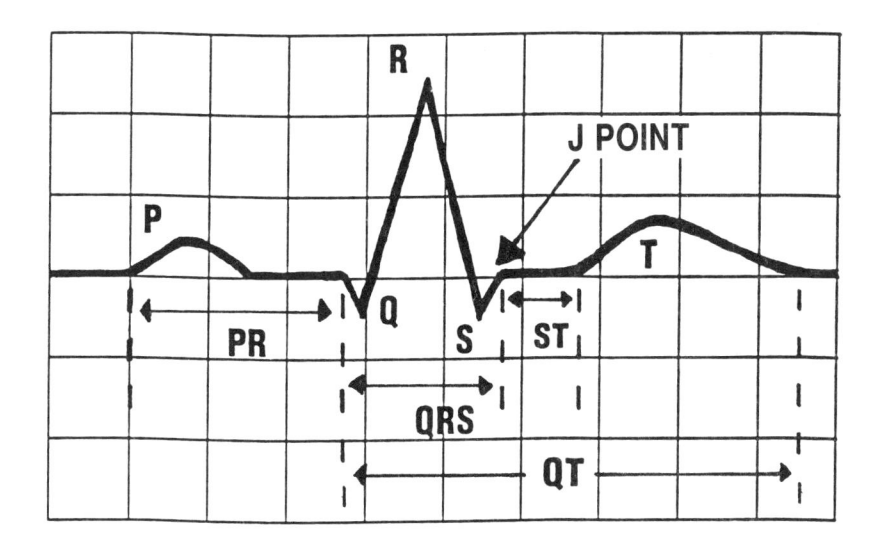

P-R INTERVAL (PRI)

The P-R interval is measured from the beginning of the P wave to the beginning of the QRS complex. It varies with heart rate, age, and the client's physique. Faster heart rates have shorter P-R intervals. Larger hearts have longer P-R intervals than small hearts. A normal P-R interval is between 0.12 to 0.20 seconds.

P-R prolongation can be a normal variation or it can be a manifestation of latent rheumatic or coronary disease.

A shortened P-R interval can happen when the electrical complex originates in the AV node or low atria. (It is also possible to have an AV nodal rhythm with no P wave.) Sometimes a shortened PRI means electrical conduction is *bypassing* the AV node; a normal P wave with a short PRI followed by a normal QRS has been associated with the tendency to develop paroxysms of tachycardia. A short PRI is also associated with hypertension.

QRS COMPLEX

On one hand the expression, "QRS complex" is a generic-type term which can describe a multitude of shapes — all of which represent ventricular depolarization. On the other hand, QRS terminology is used in a precise way to describe every twist and turn in the complex.

Rules for Naming QRS Complexes

1. The first negative (downward) deflection is a Q wave.

2. The first positive (upward) deflection is an R wave.

3. A negative deflection *that follows an R wave* is an S wave.

4. Subsequent positive deflections are called R prime (R´).

5. Subsequent negative deflections are called S prime (S´).

6. Capital and lower-case letters are assigned according to relative size of the complex. Large complexes are given capital letters while small complexes are given lower-case letters.

qRs   qR   QR   QS*

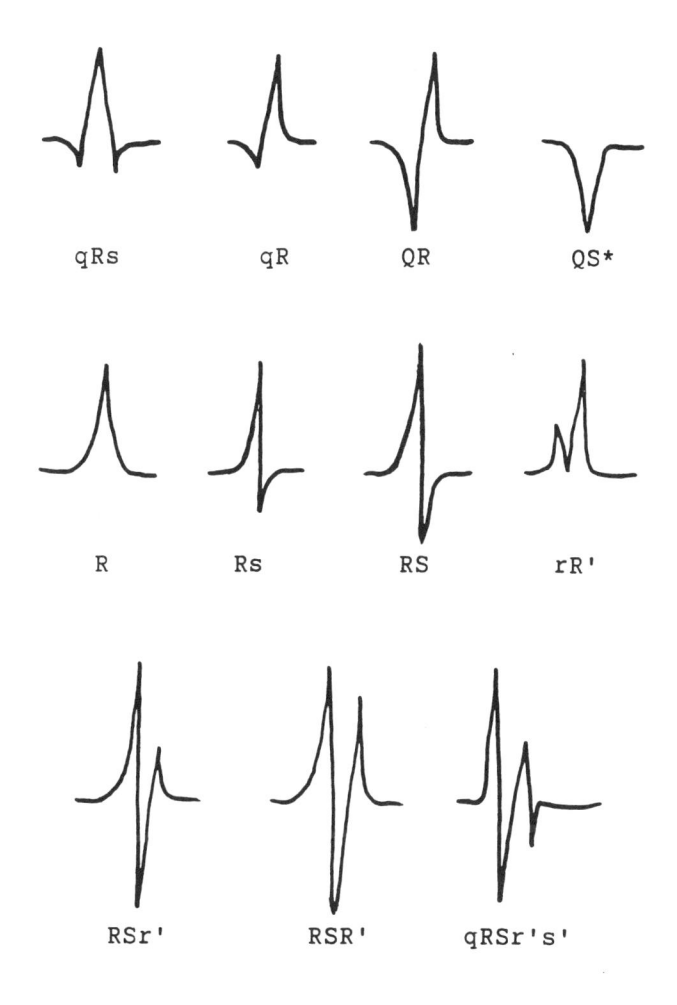

R   Rs   RS   rR'

RSr'   RSR'   qRSr's'

*A QS wave is labelled QS but we don't really know if it is just a Q wave or a QS wave.

ALL OF THESE COMPLEXES ARE CORRECTLY CALLED QRS COMPLEXES.

The *duration* of a normal QRS complex ranges from 0.05 to 0.10 second. QRS complexes with a duration greater than 0.12 second indicate abnormal intraventricular conduction.

The *amplitude* of a normal QRS complex ranges from 0.5 millivolt (5 millimeters) to 3.0 millivolts (30 millimeters) depending on the lead.

ST SEGMENT

The ST segment falls immediately after the QRS and precedes the T wave. Since the QRS complex delineates ventricular depolarization (contraction) and the T wave outlines ventricular repolarization (relaxation) — the ST segment represents the time between ventricular contraction and relaxation. The ST segment should be isoelectric, neither elevated or depressed. It should be compared with the PR segment immediately before its QRS and should be level with it. The point at which the QRS complex ends and the ST segment begins is called the J point. The ST segment is measured from the end of the QRS complex to the beginning of the T wave.

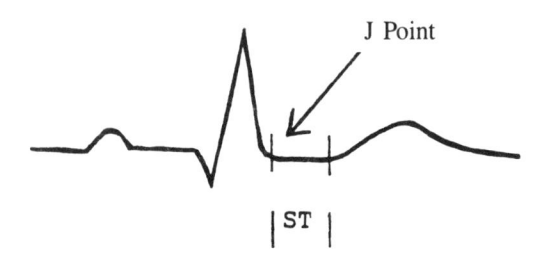

T WAVES

T waves should be gentle affairs, not sharp, not pointed, and not too tall. Rounded shapes that climb slowly from the baseline with a slightly accelerated return are normal.

QT INTERVAL

The QT interval is measured from the beginning of the QRS complex to the end of the T wave. It is often difficult to measure accurately. T waves can melt imperceptibly into the isoelectric line and sometimes T waves merge with U waves with no distinct definition of themselves. Several leads should be compared and the longest QT interval that is clearly seen should be used.

The QT interval measures the time it takes for the ventricles to contract (QRS complex) and relax (T Wave). A prolonged Q-T interval shows a delayed relaxation of the ventricles. There is the threat that the ventricles will stop relaxing altogether and will take over as the pacemaker of the heart. Prolonged QT intervals are associated with ventricular re-entry tachycardias, torsades de pointes, syncope and sudden death. Hypocalcemia, hypokalemia, and cerebral bleeds are also associated with increased QT intervals as are myocardial ischemia, infarction, and bundle branch blocks. Prolonged QT intervals can be a side effect of Class I antiarrhythmic drugs such as quinidine, procainamide and norpace.

Shortening of the QT interval is often a marker of hypercalcemia and hyperkalemia.

Upper Limits of Normal for QT Interval

Heart rate per minute	QT Interval
40	0.50
50	0.46
60	0.43
70	0.40
80	0.38
90	0.36
100	0.35
110	0.33
120	0.32
130	0.30

U WAVES

The cause of U waves is unknown. They may represent recovery of the Purkinje system or repolarization of the papillary muscles. Generally they are of the same polarity of the T waves before them. If negative U waves follow positive T waves, it often signals ischemia. Also, U waves appear more readily with bradycardia, the use of certain drugs including digoxin, epinephrine and quinidine. Hypercalcemia and hypokalemia increase their amplitude as does left ventricular hypertrophy and intracranial hemorrhage. Oh, and exercise. Plain old exercise will enlarge a U wave.

SLURRING OF THE QRS

When a QRS complex bulges outward on its upslope or downslope, it is said to be slurred.

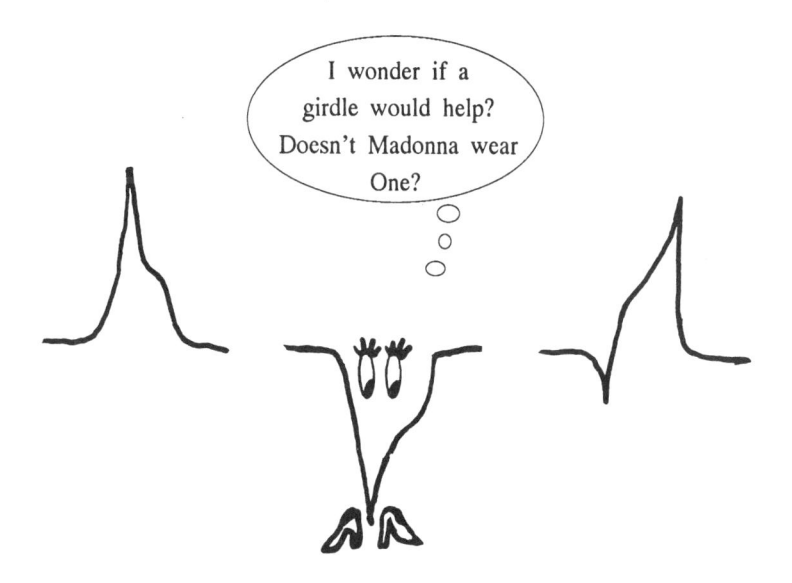

NOTCHING

Notches have sharp edges but they too disturb the crisp clean figure of a healthy QRS.

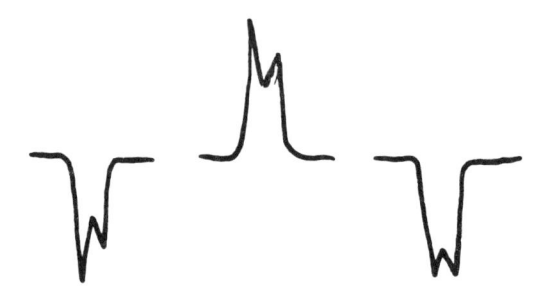

DELTA WAVES
Delta waves always occur in the beginning of the QRS. They can look like slurring or can take a more rounded shape. Often they encroach on the PR interval and shorten it. Delta waves are found in WPW (Wolf-Parkinson-White) Syndrome.

REACTION OF AN ELECTRODE

When an electrode sees an oncoming current of electricity, it draws an upright complex. When an electrode watches a wavefront fade away, it draws a negative complex. When a wave of electricity moves both toward and away from an electrode, the electrode registers a complex that is biphasic or flat.

POSITIVE COMPLEXES:
The wavefront is moving toward the electrode.

NEGATIVE COMPLEXES:
The wavefront is moving away from the electrode.

BIPHASIC COMPLEXES:
The wavefront is moving . . .
    first toward and then away

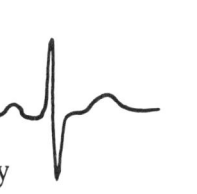

        or

first away from and then toward the electrode.

UPS AND DOWNS OF A DIPOLE

Why does a QRS complex decide to return to baseline, anyway? Let's take a positive QRS — why not keep going, say, right up to the moon?

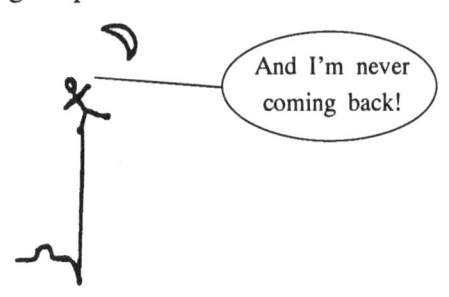

And I'm never coming back!

Actually the complex is forced to return to baseline and the point at which it turns around is very important—it's called the *intrinsic deflection*. How does the intrinsic deflection come about?

Think of the moving impulse as a pair of charges bound together, one negative and one positive. This is a dipole.

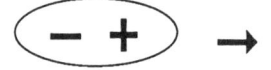

(− +) →

The positive charge is always in front, leading the way.

The Dipole Dance

1. As the dipole approaches a positive electrode two positive charges face each other and the complex swings up.

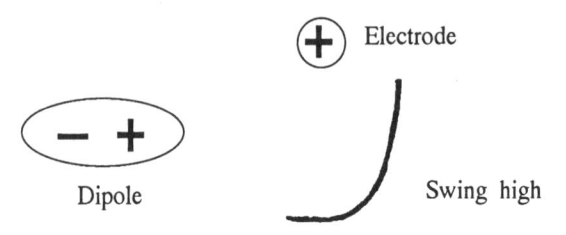

(+) Electrode

(− +) Dipole

Swing high

2. As the dipole passes directly under the electrode, there is an instantaneous change and now its negative pole faces the positive electrode.

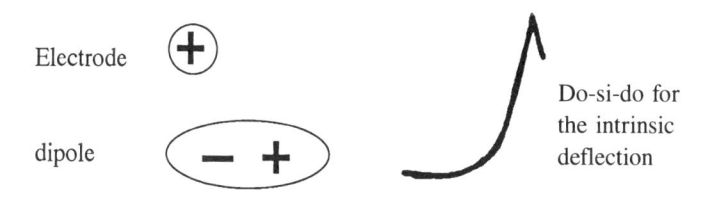

Electrode (+)

dipole (− +)

Do-si-do for the intrinsic deflection

This is the moment the complex turns around and begins a return to baseline: *the intrinsic deflection.*

3. While the negative tail faces the positive electrode, the complex will continue its negative descent.

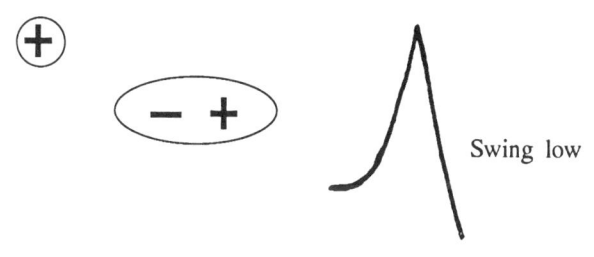

Swing low

As you can see, this is an easy dance and it just goes on and on as vectors in the heart change direction and whip around the electrodes.

In summary: When positive faces positive — swing up.

When positive faces negative — swing down,

Sweet dipole

⋯KGS JUST WANT TO HAVE FU⋯

What is normal?
Is a QRS complex wearing lingerie normal?

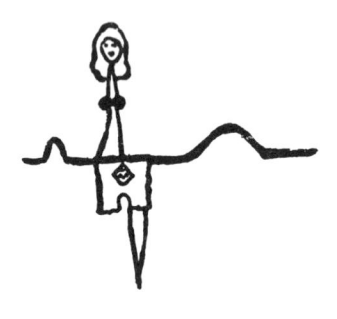

NORMAL EKG

Correct lead placement is an essential cornerstone in the interpretation of any EKG. At best a multitude of variables play a tug of war on the stylus of the EKG machine. Sometimes the heart is rotated in the chest and this will modify the shape of complexes seen. Often one cardiac condition will compete with another for expression on the EKG. For example a left bundle branch block can conceal patterns of ventricular infarction. Very often variants in the EKG are perfectly normal. Interpretation of EKGs is a subtle process and it requires correct lead placement to be worthwhile. Some authors suggest marking a patient's chest with ink to duplicate lead placement when serial EKGs are being done.

Lead by lead, here are some of the basics of a normal 12 lead EKG:

LIMB LEADS

Lead I:
    P Wave: upright

    Q Wave: small or none
        duration: should not exceed 0.03 secs
        amplitude: less than -4 mm (0.04 mV)

    QRS complex: upright
        duration: 0.05 — 0.10 secs

    T waves: upright
        amplitude: not more than 5 mm (0.5 mV)

Lead II:

P wave:	upright
Q wave:	small or none
duration:	should not exceed 0.03 secs
amplitude:	less than -4 mm (-0.4 mV)
QRS complex:	upright
	usually tallest R wave is in lead 2
duration:	0.05 — 0.10 secs
T waves:	upright
amplitude:	not above 5 mm

Lead III:

P Wave:	upright
Q wave:	small or none
duration:	should not exceed 0.04 secs
amplitude:	up to -5 mm (-0.5 mV)
QRS complex:	upright
duration	0.05 - 0.10 secs
T wave:	variable
amplitude:	not above 5 mm (0.5 mV)

Lead aVR:

P Wave	inverted
Q Wave:	QS complex is normal
QRS complex:	inverted
duration:	0.05 - 0.10 secs
T Wave:	inverted
amplitude:	not more than -5 mm (-0.5 mV)

aVL:

P Wave:	variable
Q Wave:	small or none
duration:	not more than 0.03 secs
amplitude:	less than -4 mm (-0.4 mV)
QRS complex:	upright
duration:	0.05 — 0.10 secs
T Wave:	variable
amplitude:	not more than 5 mm total

aVF:

P Wave:	upright
Q Wave:	small or none
duration:	not more than 0.03 secs
amplitude:	less than -4 mm (-0.4 mV)
QRS complex:	upright
duration:	0.05 — 0.10 secs
T Wave:	variable
amplitude:	not more than 5 mm total

Normal Q Waves

A normal Q wave in lead III can be slightly deeper and wider than in the other limb leads. A duration of up to 0.04 seconds with a depth of up to 5 mm is acceptable in a lead III. In the other limb leads the duration of a Q wave should not exceed 0.03 seconds and the depth should be less than 4 mm. Q waves are more likely to be seen in leads II, III and aVF when the axis of the heart is more vertical. When it is more horizontal, Q waves are more likely in leads I and aVL.

Amplitude of QRS

There are wide limits to the amplitude of the QRS complex. However if the total amplitude (above and below the isoelectric line) of all the QRS complexes in the limb leads is less than 5 mm, the voltage is considered abnormally low. Causes of unhealthy low voltage include hypothyroidism cardiac failure, pericardial effusion, diffuse coronary disease, emphysema, generalized edema, and obesity.

CHEST LEADS

V_1:

P Wave:	variable
R Wave:	small but present represents septal depolarization
QRS:	inverted - **right ventricular pattern**
duration:	0.05 — 0.11 secs
amplitude:	5 — 30 mm (0.5 — 3.0 mV)
T Wave:	variable
amplitude:	not more than 10 mm (1.0 mV)

V_2:

P Wave:	variable
R Wave:	larger than in V_1
QRS complex:	more negative than positive
duration:	0.05 — 0.11 secs
amplitude:	7 — 30 mm (0.7 — 3.0 mV)
T Wave:	variable
amplitude:	not more than 10 mm (1.0 mV)

V₃:

P Wave: variable

R Wave: may be less than or equal to S wave

QRS: negative or equiphasic
duration: 0.05 — 0.11 secs
amplitude: 9 — 30 mm (0.9 — 3.0 mV) total

T Wave: upright
amplitude: not more than 10 mm (1.0 mV)

V₄:

P Wave: upright

R Wave: equal to or greater than S wave

QRS: equiphasic or positive
duration: 0.05 — 0.11 secs
amplitude: 9 — 30 mm (0.9 — 3.0 mV)

T Wave: upright
amplitude: not more than 10 mm (1.0 mV)

V₅:

P Wave: upright

Q Wave: small but present

QRS: upright
duration: 0.05 — 0.11 secs
amplitude: 7 — 30 mm (0.7 — 3.0 mV)

T Wave: upright
amplitude: not more than 10 mm (1.0 mV)

V_6:

P Wave: variable

Q Wave: small but present

QRS: positive **(left ventricular pattern)**
  duration: 0.05 — 0.11 secs
  amplitude: 5 — 30 mm (0.5 — 3.0 mV)

T Wave: positive
  amplitude: not more than 10 mm (1.0 mV)

NORMAL COMPLEXES IN THE V LEADS

Arrows represent sequence of ventricular depolarization

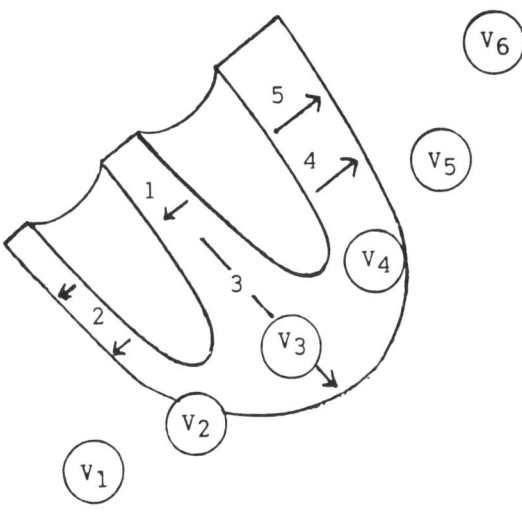

The small but significant R wave in V1 expresses depolarization of the ventricular *septum*. You can see the wave of electricity *first* travelling across the septum toward the electrode at V_1. The impulse continues on and quickly completes its journey across the thin wall of the right ventricle. It takes longer for the vector to penetrate the thick muscular wall of the left ventricle but as it finally does, a large S wave is seen. This is called a ***right ventricular pattern*** because the electrode sits near the right ventricle. Despite the name of this pattern, the S wave sketches out the depolarization of the powerful left ventricle, while the events of the right ventricle are lost in the shadows.

Although depolarization is portrayed here in a two dimensional plane, please remember all these electrical happenings take place in three dimensions. As the initial wavefront moves across the septum and through the right ventricle, it is moving *anteriorly* as well as left to right. The right ventricle lies toward the front of the chest while the left ventricle is behind it. Another point to keep in mind is that the septum is a thick muscular wall that is really part of the left ventricle.

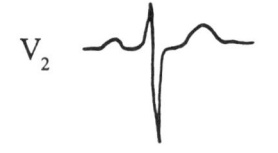

V_2 — The R wave should grow a little in V_2. It is important to look for *R wave progression* in the V leads. It shows that the septum is alive and well and conducting electricity. If you don't see an R wave here, be suspicious of a septal infarct. Other causes of poor R wave progression include left ventricular hypertrophy, emphysema, and left bundle branch block.

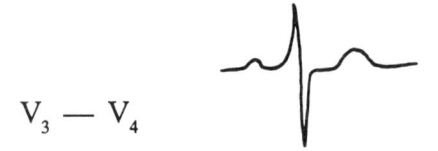

$V_3 — V_4$ *Zone of Transition*

Look for an equiphasic complex (equally positive and negative) in V_3 or V_4. This makes sense if you look at the vectors as they move both toward and away from the electrodes there.

If this transition comes *early* it may signify right ventricular hypertrophy. The right ventricle can hold onto a wave longer if it wall is thicker. This would be considered *anterior axis deviation.* Conversely a *late* transition may represent left ventricular hypertrophy as the wave would take longer to transverse an enlarged muscle to finally emerge at the skin. This would be considered *posterior axis deviation.** But then ... early and late transition can just be a normal variant. Don't you just love it?

V_5 & V_6 In these leads we see a small q wave represent septal depolarization as the initial vector moves away from the electrodes at V_5 and V_6. The large R wave is left ventricular activation. The pattern at V_6 is called a *left ventricular pattern* because its electrode perches near the left ventricle.

---

* This theory has not been supported by anatomic correlation study.

AXIS DEVIATION

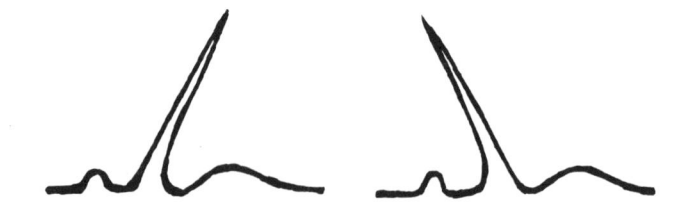

DETERMINATION OF AXIS

Remember the hexaxial reference system.

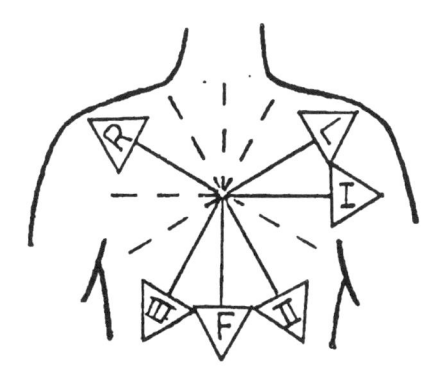

YEAH

Hexaxial reference is used in calculating the axis of the heart. Each of the arcs made in the circle of leads is assigned 30 degrees and axes can be assigned precise mathematical orientations. It *is* important to do this. For example a shift to the right of an axis could indicate a pulmonary embolus. This text, however, does not go into instruction on this calculation. Many of the texts in our bibliography do.

We like a very simple method to determine a rough calculation of the axis that takes less than two minutes to do.

Two-Minute, Two-Lead Method for Axis Determination

The mean cardiac vector is downward from right to left so a normal axis follows the same direction. How can we tell if the axis is not normal?

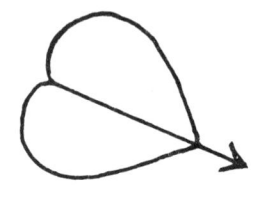

If we concentrate on leads *I* and *aVF*, we see that these two leads lie on the perimeter of normal axis. If the QRS is *upright* in both of these leads, the axis of the heart is *normal*. (Lead II lies in the center of normal axis and this is the reason that the tallest R wave is usually in lead II.)

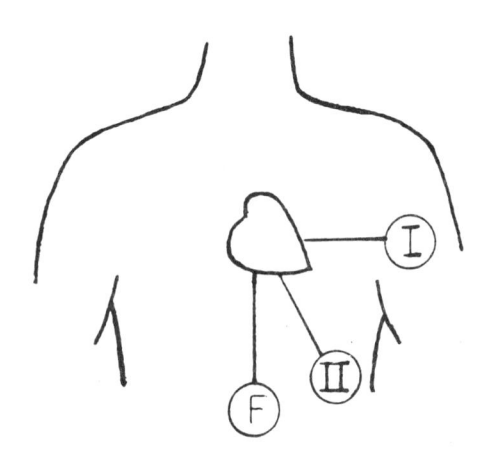

We can see right or left axis deviation by using these same two leads:

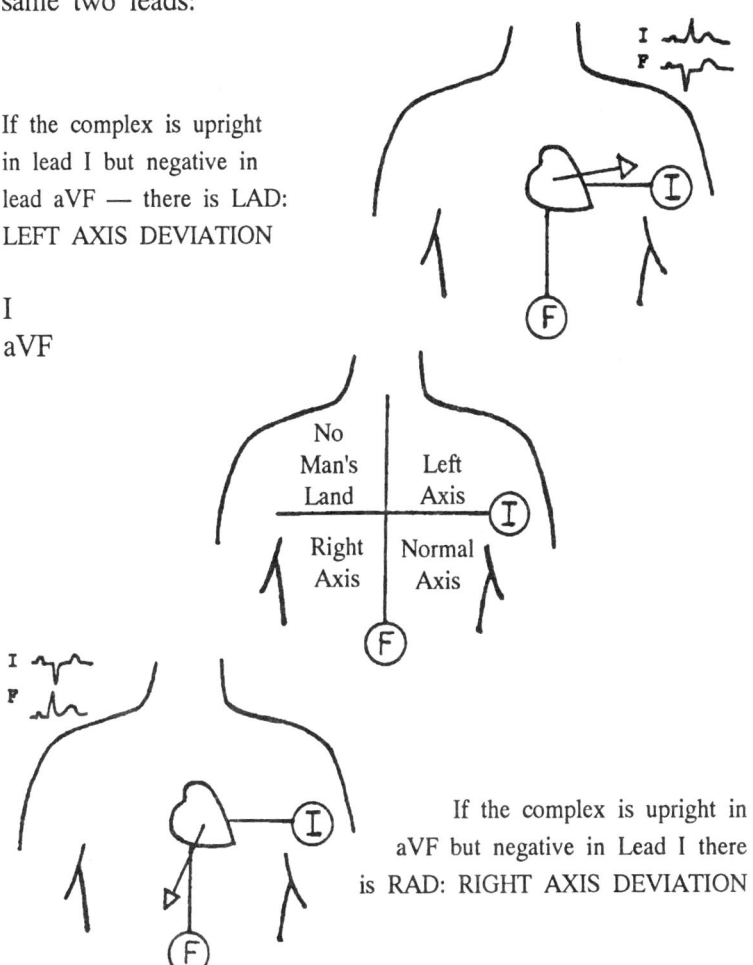

If the complex is upright in lead I but negative in lead aVF — there is LAD: LEFT AXIS DEVIATION

I
aVF

If the complex is upright in aVF but negative in Lead I there is RAD: RIGHT AXIS DEVIATION

If the complexes are *negative* in both leads I and *aVF* — there is an indeterminate or unknown axis. Some experts believe negative complexes in both these leads signifies an extreme right axis. Some call it a ride to *No Mans Land*.

57

Two Lead Method For Determining Axis Deviation

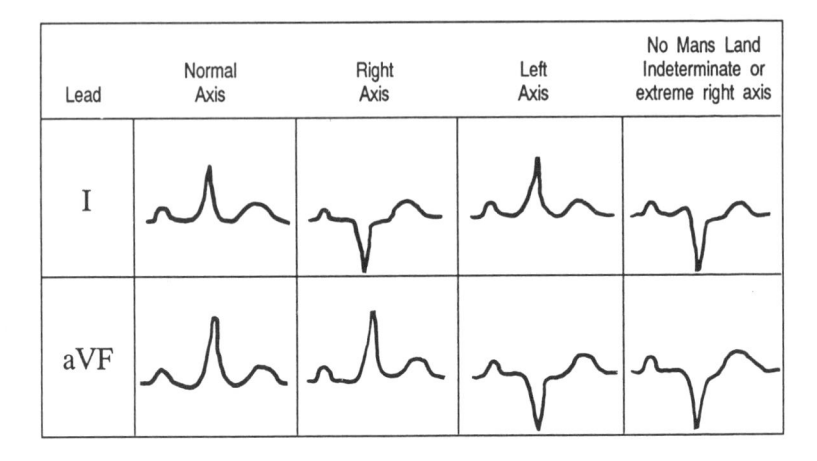

Lead	Normal Axis	Right Axis	Left Axis	No Mans Land Indeterminate or extreme right axis
I	⋀	⋁	⋀	⋁
aVF	⋀	⋀	⋁	⋁

Causes of Axis Deviation

Right	Left
Normal Variation	Normal Variation
Inspiration	Exhalation
Right Ventricular Hypertrophy	Left Ventricular Hypertrophy
*Right Bundle Branch Block	*Left Bundle Branch Block
Left Posterior Hemiblock	Left Anterior Hemiblock
Lateral Infarction	Inferior Infarction
Dextrocardia	Pregnancy
Pulmonary Embolism	Obesity

*When right bundle branch block is associated with right axis deviation, usually left posterior hemiblock and/or right ventricular hypertrophy is involved.

*Left bundle branch block with left axis deviation is usually indicative of left ventricular dysfunction.

Several conditions can cause axis deviation to the left or right and these include emphysema, ventricular ectopic rhythms and Wolf-Parkinson-White syndrome.

WITHIN NORMAL LIMITS

ST Segments: ST segments should curve gently into the upslope of the T waves

T Waves: Should be mild-mannered with gradual upslopes that have a slightly steeper return to the baseline

The height of T waves should not exceed 5 mm in limb leads or 10 mm in precordial leads

Physiological Q Waves: Small narrow Q waves

Vertical heart Q waves in II, III, aVF
Horizontal heart Q waves in I & aVL

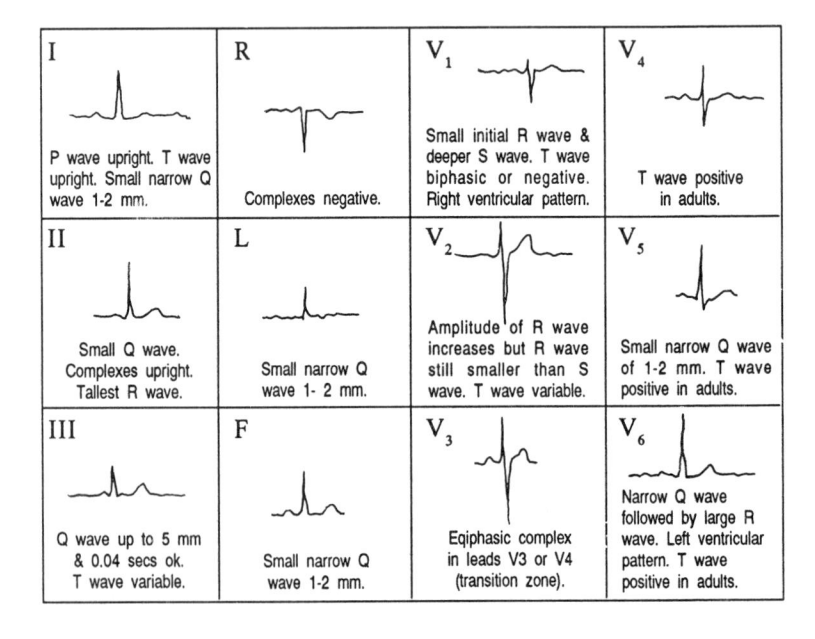

I	R	V_1	V_4
P wave upright. T wave upright. Small narrow Q wave 1-2 mm.	Complexes negative.	Small initial R wave & deeper S wave. T wave biphasic or negative. Right ventricular pattern.	T wave positive in adults.
II	L	V_2	V_5
Small Q wave. Complexes upright. Tallest R wave.	Small narrow Q wave 1- 2 mm.	Amplitude of R wave increases but R wave still smaller than S wave. T wave variable.	Small narrow Q wave of 1-2 mm. T wave positive in adults.
III	F	V_3	V_6
Q wave up to 5 mm & 0.04 secs ok. T wave variable.	Small narrow Q wave 1-2 mm.	Eqiphasic complex in leads V3 or V4 (transition zone).	Narrow Q wave followed by large R wave. Left ventricular pattern. T wave positive in adults.

SECTION TWO

MYOCARDIAL INFARCTION

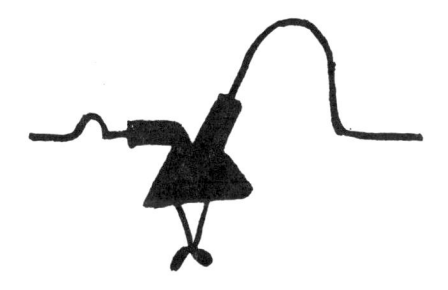

No, I haven't been working out my left arm. It's just a little injury. The important thing is — do you like the dress?

The Fairytale Continues . . .

The Real Thing

Prince Ischemia's chauffeur parked his silver mercedes in his spotless white garage. Outside a number of ambulances and cars were parked all over the grounds of the fabubrick castle. There was alot of packages to carry, as the prince had been shopping.

Prince Ischemia was delivered to the main entrance and he raced through its gleaming marble doors, shouting, "What's going on?" to a multitude of doctors, nurses, and hospital types that definitely seemed out of place here.

"Your majesty," his secretary appeared out of the crowd. "Your sister's had a heart attack! I'll take you right to her."

What a commotion was being made. Word had leaked out and subjects sent song-grams and flowers. Nurses hovered over his sister, taking blood pressures and fussing with electrodes hooked to wires, hooked to ringing monitors. The prince was intrigued by the equipment but his sister looked just great to him. Dr. Finebeat was at her bedside, pushing a tube of medicine into one of her many IVs. The exhausted cardiologist had just nicknamed her Princess Infarction. It was obvious to everyone in the room that her newly arrived brother was upset.

The prince had always been jealous of his sister and this fanned those green flames in a cruel and unrelenting way.

"Hi sister," he said dully

"Prince, thank you for coming to see me in my suite. Don't worry about me — I'll be fine."

"I'm sure you will be," said the prince, glaring at Dr. Finebeat. "In fact, I must say I'm somewhat surprised no one's concerned about me. Did you know that occasionally I have inverted T waves in my inferior leads. And a right-sided EKG I had just last week showed ST depression in V_3R.

"Oh, not-to-worry," assured the Princess. "Remember when the wicked witch turned me into a hairless dog? Well, a mad scientist in her employment cut open my chest and tied off a coronary artery. Immediately my EKG showed inverted T waves. It was serious but reversible. When the crazy scientist untied the ligature, the T waves righted themselves in no time at all."

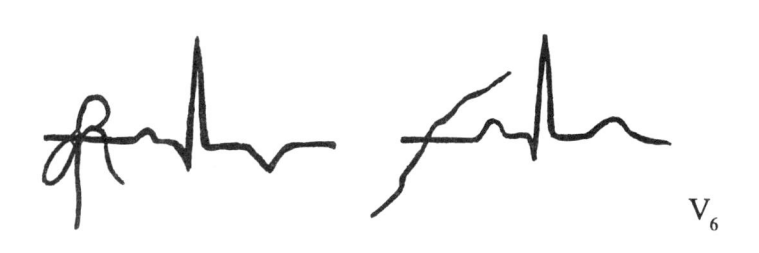

V_6

"Don't tell me not to worry about my EKG," Ischemia stamped a long foot encased in a brand new shoe of the finest leather. He tore through his pockets looking for his favorite EKG. Look at my ST segments — they're depressed!

"But mine," said Infarction, "are elevated."

"Not every much," accused her seething brother.

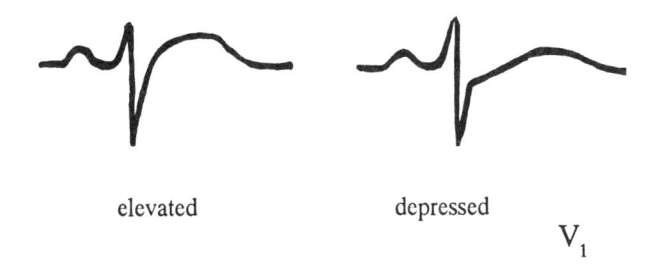

elevated   depressed

V_1

"It's not the size that matters," the princess said gently. "its the shape."

"You're making that up." sneered the Prince.

At this time an eaves-dropping hospital nurse who had been charting frenziedly dressed in iridescent pink and lavender scrubs checked her care plan and saw it was clearly time to implement a nursing action. Her name was Lucina. Lucina tiptoed over to the battling royalties.

"Your majesties," Lucina said in a gentle tone, "Please don't argue. You know," she sighed deeply, "People say critical care personnel take care of the nearly dead, the newly dead, *and the very very dead. Indeed, Princess Infarction's EKG shows what we call tombstone T's. And she's absolutely right about size and shape. It isn't so much the size of her ST elevations but the ugly coved shape they have that is so ominous.*

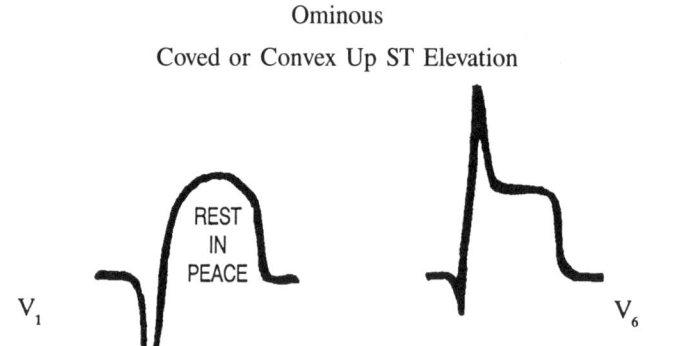

Ominous
Coved or Convex Up ST Elevation

V_1 REST IN PEACE V_6

"What about my inverted T waves and ST segment depression!" screamed Ischemia.

"I believe Dr. Finebeat prescribed some nitroglycerin sublingual for you," Lucina was already scurrying toward the medicine cabinet. "And you really should get some rest."

MYOCARDIAL INFARCTION

COGNITIVE OBJECTIVES

* Identify the main coronary arteries and the muscles they perfuse.
* Describe the evolution of an MI.
* Describe the characteristics of a normal ST segment and T wave.
* Identify three classic EKG changes in an acute MI.
* Identify what to look for in the indicative and reciprocal leads.
* Identify the indicative and reciprocal leads for the anterior wall, the inferior wall and the lateral wall.
* Describe how to look for EKG changes associated with a posterior wall MI.
* Describe how to look for a right ventricular MI.
* Describe the EKG changes seen in acute pericarditis.

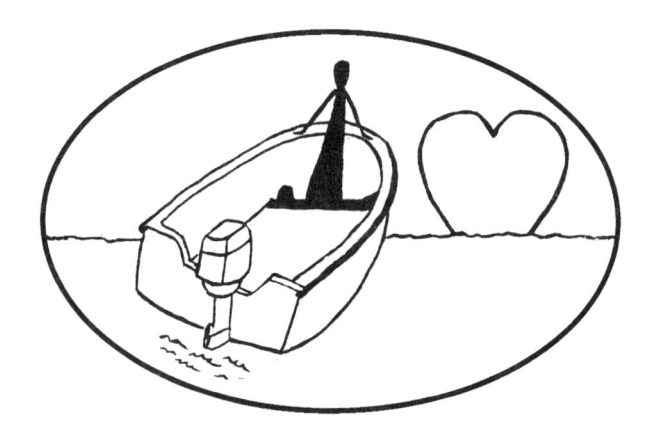

THE CORONARY ARTERIES

THE CORONARY ARTERIES

There are two eminent arteries that bestow a blood supply to the myocardium — the *left coronary artery* and the *right coronary artery*. At the sinuses of Valsalva, which are located in the aorta behind the cusp of the aortic valve, they originate from small openings called ostia and branch out to nourish the heart. The left coronary artery (or left *main* coronary artery) usually perfuses most of the left atrium and left ventricle while the right coronary artery perfuses the right atrium and right ventricle. Not all hearts are the same, however, and a great deal of variation exists from one individual to the next.

The left coronary artery divides almost immediately into two major branches: the *left anterior descending artery* and the *left circumflex artery*. In some hearts a third branch is sandwiched between these two and it is called the *ramus intermedius artery*.

Left Anterior Descending Artery (LAD):
The LAD delivers blood to the left ventricular free wall. Additionally several branches of the LAD called *septal perforating arteries* supply the anterior two thirds of the interventricular septum — in which nestles the main trunk of the right bundle branch and both major fasicles of the left bundle

1. Left main
2. Right coronary
3. Circumflex
4. Left anterior descending
5. Septal perforators
6. Diagonals

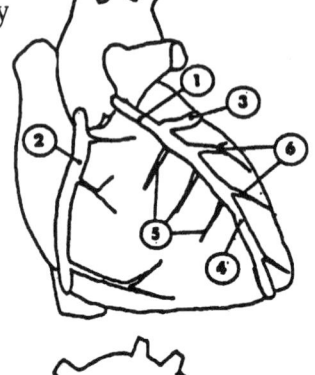

7. Obtuse marginals
8. Ramus intermedius

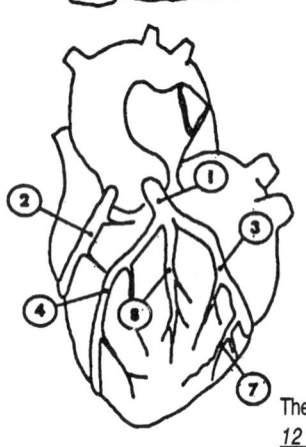

9. Posterior descending
10. AV nodal
11. Septal perforators

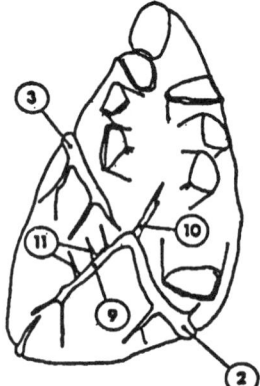

The Coronary Arteries from *12 Lead ECG Interpretation: A Self-Assessment Approach* by Zainul Abedin, MD, FACC FRCP(C) and Robert Connor, RN, CCRN. Reprinted with permission of the authors and W.B. Saunders, Philadelphia.

branch. Other branches of the LAD called *diagonal arteries* furnish blood to the anteriolateral wall of the left ventricle. Occlusion of the LAD results in an *anterior wall infarction*. Interventricular conduction disturbances are likely if occlusion of the LAD occurs high enough to cut off circulation to the septum.

Left Circumflex Artery: The left circumflex artery gives its blood to the lateral wall of the left ventricle. In about ten percent of hearts, the left circumflex slips under the bottom of the heart to give birth to the posterior descending artery. Occlusion of the circumflex artery results in *lateral wall infarction*. When the circumflex artery fathers the posterior descending artery, occlusion of the circumflex may create a posterior wall infarction as well.

Right Coronary Artery (RCA): The RCA travels down the right side of the heart offering blood to the right atrium and right ventricle. In *ninety percent* of hearts, the RCA gives rise to the *posterior descending artery*. The posterior descending artery has *septal perforating branches* that perfuse the posterior one-third of the interventricular septum. Right and left septal perforating arteries anastomose providing essential collateral circulation. Occlusion of the RCA results in *inferior wall infarction and/or posterior wall infarction*.

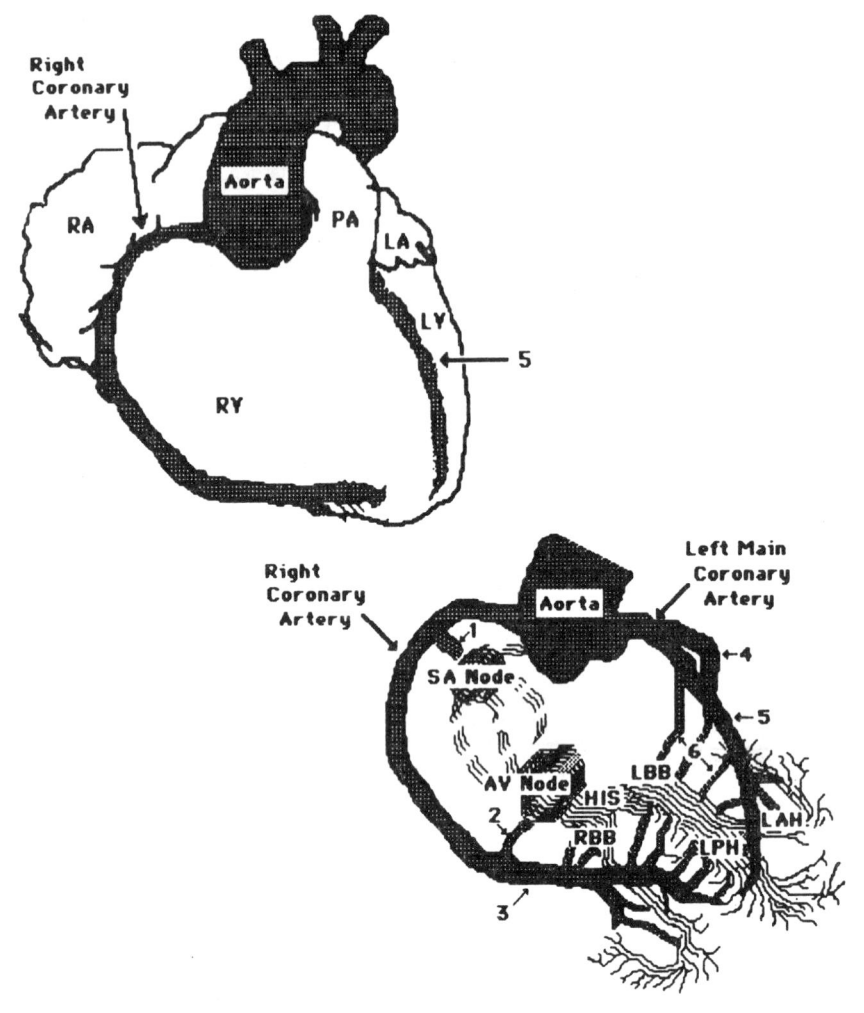

The heart and the coronary circulation. RA - Right atrium. LA - Left atrium. RV - Right ventricle. LV - Left ventricle. PA - Pulmonary artery. 1 - SA nodal artery. 2 - AV nodal artery. 3 - Posterior descending artery. 4 - Circumflex artery. 5 - Left anterior descending artery. 6 - Septal perforating arteries. *From Clinical Electrocardiography by Ken Grauer, MD and R. Whitney Curry Jr., MD. A Medical Economics Book. Reprinted with permission from Blackwell Scientific Publications in Cambridge, Massachusetts. 1987*

Dominance and the Posterior Descending Artery

When the left circumflex artery supplies the posterior descending artery the heart is said to be "left dominant." When the right coronary artery supplies the posterior descending artery the heart is considered to be "right dominant" (which is the case in most people).

The term "dominant" can be confusing. The left coronary artery is larger and perfuses more of the heart than the right coronary artery although most people are called "right dominant." *Dominance* is just a term that describes the terminal portion of the right coronary artery versus the terminal portion of the left circumflex artery.

The Nodes: In fifty-five percent of hearts a branch of the RCA forms the *sinus node artery* which perfuses the sinus node. In forty-five percent of hearts, the left circumflex forms the sinus node artery.

In ninety percent of hearts a branch of the RCA forms the *atrioventricular nodal artery* which perfuses the atrioventricular node. In ten percent of hearts the left circumflex forms the AV nodal artery.

Enough background, right? As in RCA,

left descending,

circumflex.

Easy.

THE LANDSCAPE OF MYOCARDIAL INFARCTION

IMAGES OF ISCHEMIA, INJURY & NECROSIS

If we could place tiny electrodes directly on the throbbing, infarcting hearts of our clients, we would see pure patterns of ischemia (inverted T waves), injury (ST elevation), and necrosis (Q waves). These patterns would correspond to zones on the heart of the same.

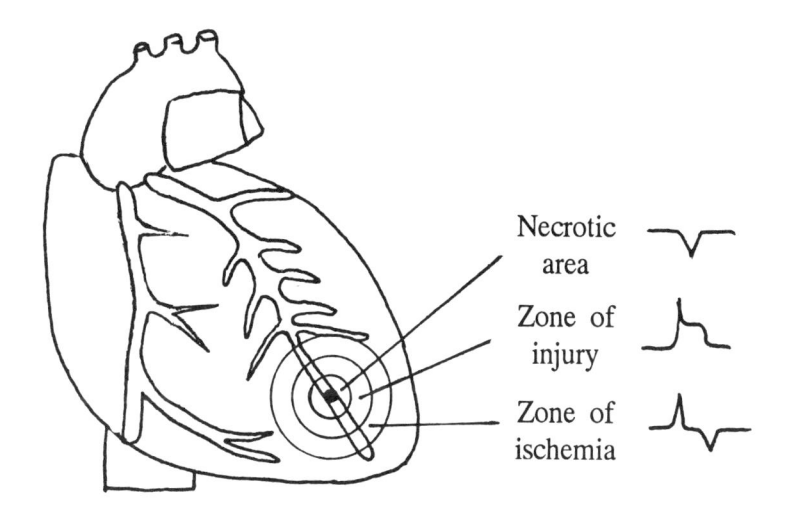

Necrotic area

Zone of injury

Zone of ischemia

Mad scientists have done this to "experimental" hearts of dogs and other little animals.

Since the electrodes we usually get to use are an inch or two away from pure patterns, we see a composite picture of all of them.

Composite Picture of
a Q Wave, ST Elevation and an Inverted T Wave

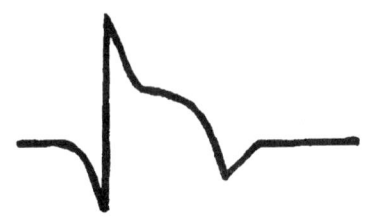

ISCHEMIA
T Wave Inversion and/or ST Depression

Symmetrical "arrowhead" T wave inversion in a lead which normally has an upright T wave is a hallmark of ischemia. The reason inverted arrowhead T waves form is unknown. Some believe that during ischemia negative charges may leak across the cell membrane and interfere with the cell's ability to repolarize.

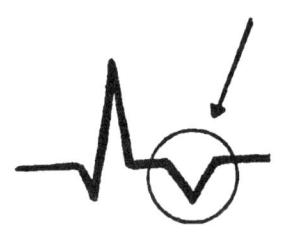

Not all T wave inversion is due to ischemia. Such cardiac conditions as bundle branch block, ventricular hypertrophy, and pericarditis can cause it. A number of conditions unrelated to the heart including electrolyte disorders, shock and changes in position can too. But T wave inversion caused by conditions other than ischemia is usually *a*symmetrical — no arrowheads.

ST Segment Depression

Another classic marker of ischemia is ST segment depression. Often you will see this in combination with a sharp angle at the junction of the ST segment and the T wave.

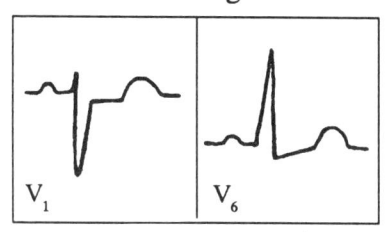

INJURY
ST Elevation

No one knows for sure why cardiac injury paints a pattern of ST elevation. If negative charges do leak across a cell's membrane when it is hurt, there would be a loss of resting membrane potential (the charge of the cell's interior as opposed to the charge across the membrane in the extracellular fluid).* This loss in resting membrane potential could depress the baseline of the EKG (Q-T segment) which would make the ST segment look elevated.

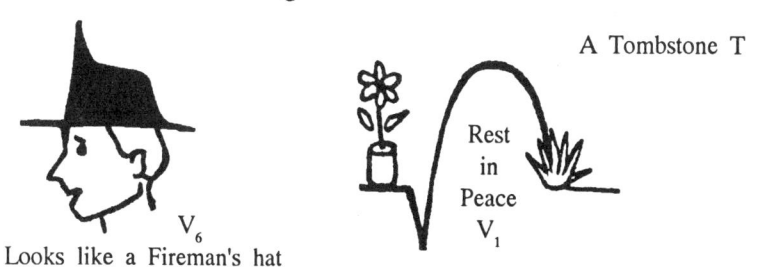

A Tombstone T

V_6
Looks like a Fireman's hat

Rest in Peace
V_1

* For an explanation of a resting membrane potential, see pages in Appendix.

Now, there are ST elevations and ... ST elevations. You must look closely at the *shape* of them. The ST elevations that are deadly are *coved* or convex up. You could say they turn an unsmiling face to the world. The *other* type of ST elevations — the smiling ones — are not always ominous. Sometimes they're just a normal variant — a result of early repolarization. Sometimes they're a result of pericarditis. *A smiling ST elevation is not an infarcting ST elevation.*

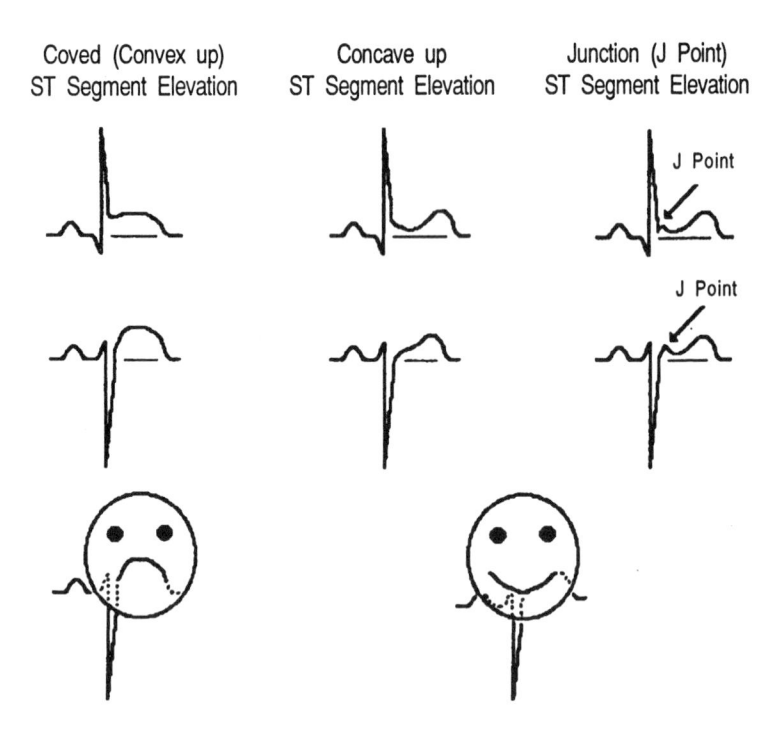

Coved (Convex up) ST Segment Elevation	Concave up ST Segment Elevation	Junction (J Point) ST Segment Elevation

Reprinted with permission from Blackwell Scientific Publications from Clinical Electrography, A Primary Care Approach by Ken Grauer, MD and R. Whitney Curry Jr. M.D. 1987

NECROSIS
Q Waves

Q waves show dead tissue — necrosis. This makes perfect sense. Dead tissue can't conduct electrical impulses and so the wavefront moves away from it. Q waves must be deep or wide or both to be significant. If a Q wave is larger than 0.04 seconds (one baby box) or as deep as 25% of the R wave, it is suspicious.

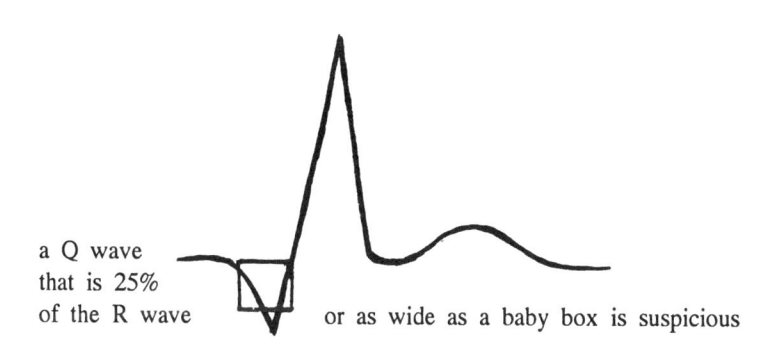

a Q wave that is 25% of the R wave   or as wide as a baby box is suspicious

Sometimes the Q wave incurred with an infarction will stay with a person a lifetime. Other times the Q wave will shrink and not look as malevolent as it once did. And sometimes the Q wave of an MI will disappear over time altogether.

Once it was thought that an infarction had to involve the entire thickness of the cardiac wall to produce a Q wave. Hand-in-hand with this idea went the reasoning that if an MI didn't produce a Q wave, it didn't pierce the entire wall. Non Q-wave infarctions were called sub-endocardial (part-of-the-wall-only) infarctions. This thinking is no longer fashionable.

Now it is known that if the heart is rotated in the chest, it can endure an MI without ever producing a Q wave. Are such MIs called rotated MIs? No — they are called non Q-wave MIs. How can we be wrong with that name? *Non Q-wave MIs* are diagnosed with the client's history, ST elevation and T wave inversion — and don't forget the cardiac enzymes.

INDICATIVE AND RECIPROCAL LEADS

Indicative leads face the wall of injury and display the signs of injury and/or infarction. Reciprocal leads are distant from the injury and reflect, in an upside-down, mirror image the changes seen in indicative leads. These reciprocal changes are the signs of ischemia.

ST elevation in an indicative lead is seen as

ST depression in a reciprocal lead.

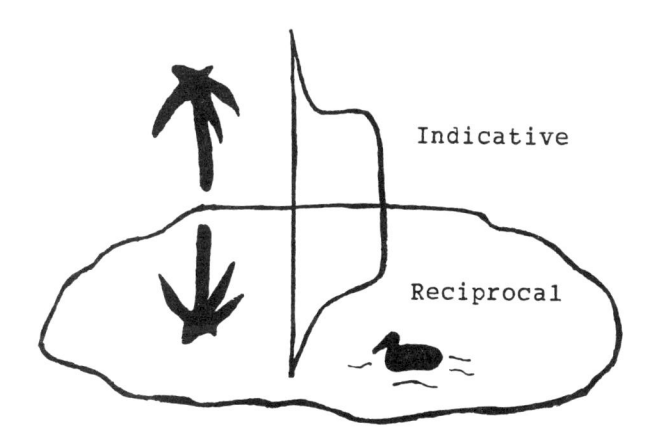

ST elevation is the mark of injury.

ST depression is a reciprocal change.

Note, however, that ST depression can be a sign of simple ischemia. *It doesn't have to be a reciprocal change* — it can be a change in its own right.

EVOLUTION OF AN MI

Like many things in this world, an MI has its ages and stages — and here they manifest themselves in the lines of squiggles of a 12-lead EKG. In the infant (or hyperacute) stage, there are abnormally tall T waves. Some people wonder if potassium isn't leaking out of the cell at this time because hyperkalemia can do this, too.

Next we see coved ST segment elevation in the indicative leads, with T wave inversion and a beginning Q wave.

In the third stage, the ST segment returns to baseline but the Q wave and T wave invasion persist. In fact, the T wave inversion deepens.

Finally the T wave assumes a normal shape. The ST segment may look a little flattened. Usually a Q wave remains.

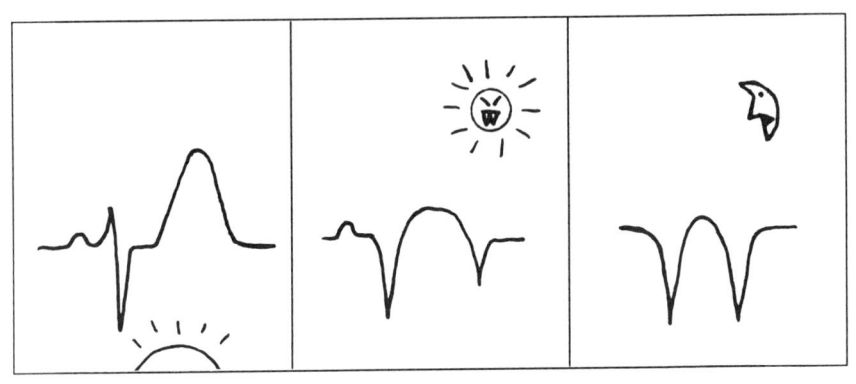

Evolution of Anteroseptal Wall MI in V_3

Evolution Of Inferior Wall MI

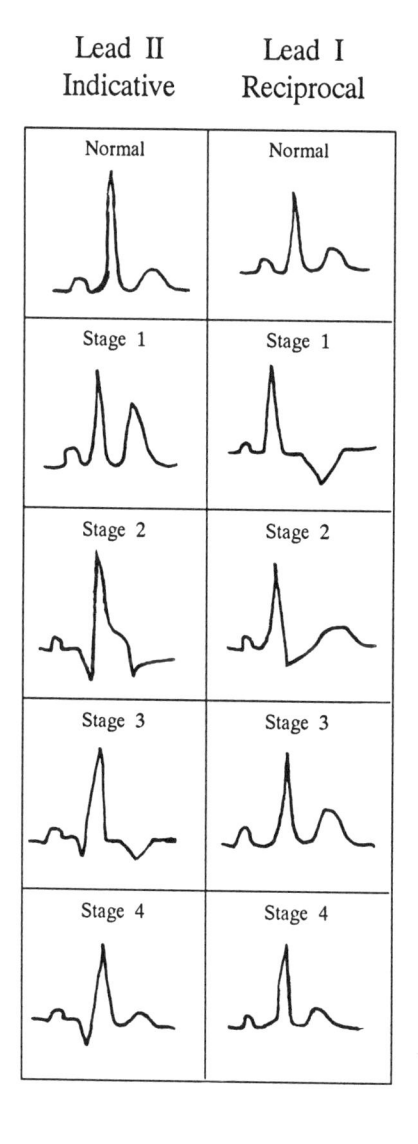

Lead II Indicative	Lead I Reciprocal
Normal	Normal
Stage 1	Stage 1
Stage 2	Stage 2
Stage 3	Stage 3
Stage 4	Stage 4

INFARCTION, WALL TO WALL

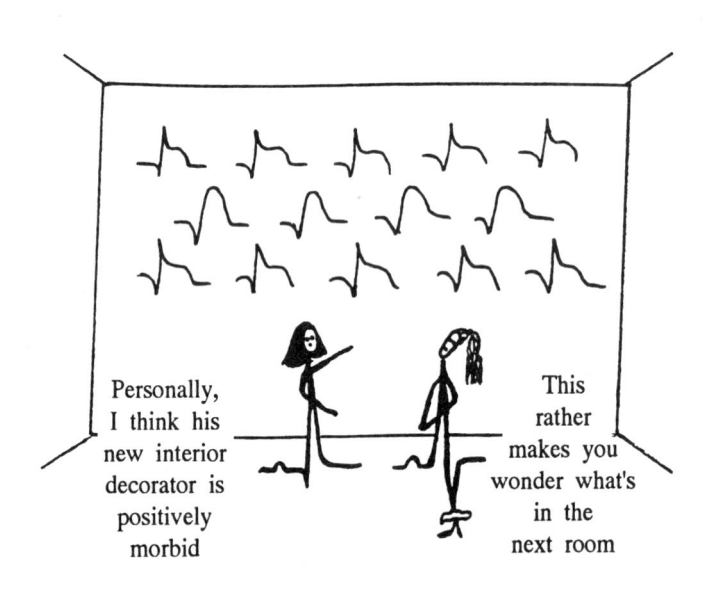

Personally, I think his new interior decorator is positively morbid

This rather makes you wonder what's in the next room

ANTERIOR WALL MI

Occlusion of the Widow-maker, sometimes called the Artery of Sudden Death, sometimes called the *left anterior descending artery,* is the culprit in anterior wall infarction. Coved ST segment elevation, T wave inversion and Q waves will be seen in the precordial leads and these are indicative changes. Reciprocal changes are found in leads II, III and aVF and here you would see ST depression.

The sequela of anterior wall infarctions is often lethal. A large area of the heart muscle can be involved and for this reason, *cardiogenic shock* is more likely with anterior wall infarction than with necrosis in the other walls. *Conduction defects* tend to be serious and include bundle branch blocks, Mobitz II 2° AV block and third degree heart block. *Sympathetic hyperactivity* is common with its sinus tachycardia and/or hypertension.

If there is a septal infarction involved as well, the R waves will be missing in V_1 and V_2. A *pure septal infarction* — without infarction of the left ventricular free wall — will show QS complexes in V_1 and V_2. ST elevation will not be evident.

LATERAL WALL INFARCTION

Occlusion of the *circumflex* causes lateral wall infarction. ST elevation, inverted T waves and Q waves are seen in leads I, aVL, V_5 and V_6. Sometimes ST depression can be seen in V_1. A drop in the QRS amplitude in I, aVL, V_5 and V_6 can indicate a lateral wall MI. Conduction defects are rare. Lateral wall infarctions usually result from extension of anterior or inferior wall infarction.

INFERIOR WALL INFARCTION

Occlusion of the *right coronary artery* is usually the cause of inferior wall infarction. ST elevation, inverted T waves and Q waves will be seen in leads II, III, and aVF with ST depression in leads I and aVL. Occasionally, occlusion of the left circumflex causes inferior wall infarction. When this is the case, there will be ST elevation in one or more of the lateral leads (aVL V_5 and V_6) with no reciprocal change in lead I.

Conduction defects are usually transient and include 1° AV block and Mobitz I. *Parasympathetic hyperactivity* is common with bradyarrythmias and hypotension frequently seen. Vagal maneuvers such as straining can precipitate atrioventricular block which is why colace is an official drug of the unit.

POSTERIOR WALL INFARCTION

Suspect a posterior wall infarct when tall R waves are present in V_1 or V_2 with ST depression right next to them. There are no indicative leads for the posterior wall and what you are looking at are reciprocal changes. You can do the famous "mirror test."

MIRROR TEST FOR POSTERIOR WALL INFARCTION

1. Take the EKG, flip it over to the unprinted side and turn it upside down. Now the tall "R" waves are deep Q waves and ST depression becomes ST elevation.

That's it. It's an easy one step test — just look at the images in V_1, V_2, and V_3 as if they were upside down and backwards.

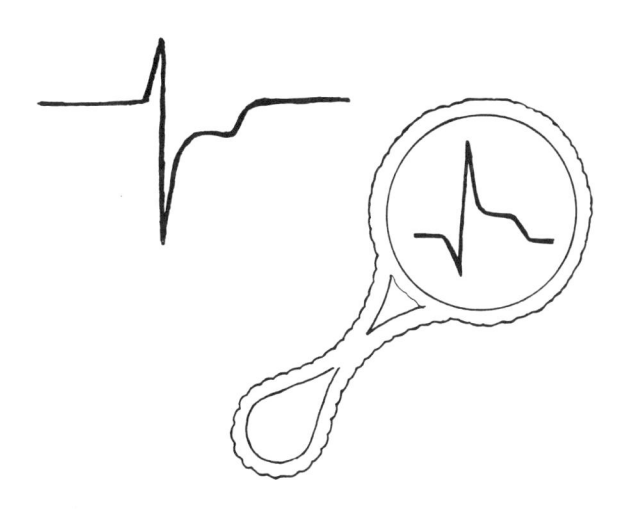

Blockage of the *posterior descending artery* will cause a posterior wall infarction. Posterior wall infarctions are particularly common with inferior wall infarctions. The right coronary artery supplies the inferior wall and usually gives rise to the posterior descending artery. Sometimes the left circumflex fathers the posterior descending artery.

RIGHT VENTRICULAR INFARCTION

Although right ventricular infarction can present alone, it is usually associated with inferior wall infarction. It is the product of an occlusion in the *right coronary artery.* Since the right ventricle is not well represented on a standard left-sided EKG — try looking at it this way:

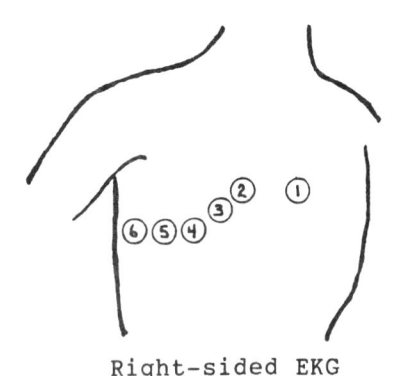

Right-sided EKG

In right ventricular infarction ST elevation will be apparent in right-sided V leads. Other signs and symptoms to look for include:

1. Hypotension
2. Jugular venous distension
3. Ventricular gallop: S3
4. Summation gallop: S3 + S4
5. Clear lungs
6. Kussmaul's sign
7. Increase in right atrial pressure and increase in CVP

The damaged right ventricle cannot pump enough blood during systole. Therefore less blood enters the left ventricle, resulting in decreased blood pressure and decreased cardiac output. This is a great climate for shock.

As the heart tries to compensate by increasing its rate, the tachycardia and decreased filling time reduce the cardiac output even further. This patient needs fluids to stretch the stiff right ventricle into doing its job.

A NORMAL RIGHT-SIDED EKG

Here is an example of a normal right-sided EKG. The complex in the V leads get smaller and smaller as the wavefront of current becomes more distant to the monitoring electrodes. The important thing is that there is *no ST elevation* in the V leads and an R wave is present in V_1R and V_2R. Also there are *no Q waves in the V leads.*

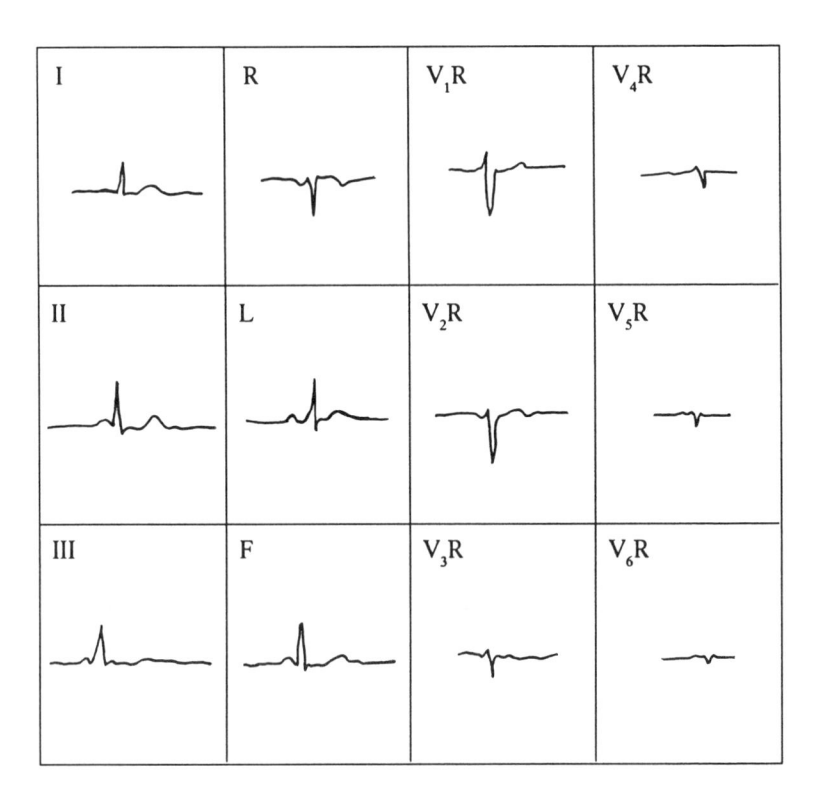

I	R	V_1R	V_4R
II	L	V_2R	V_5R
III	F	V_3R	V_6R

ATRIAL INFARCTION

When atrial arrythmias develop in the midst of a ventricular infarction — suspect an atrial infarction. Look for abnormal P wave contours and P-R segment displacement.

OH NO!! Where is my zit cream? I have a date tonight with the nicest QRS in V1. And look at my PR segment!

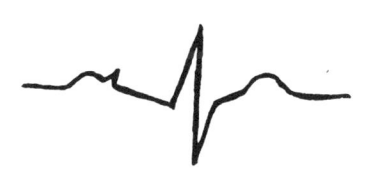

ANTERIOR WALL MI

Indicative Leads: I, aVL, V_1 - V_4

Reciprocal Leads: II, III, aVF

Arterial Perfusion: Left Anterior Descending
(Widow-maker or Artery of Sudden Death)

Potential Complications:
Sympathetic Hyperactivity
Sinus Tachycardia (may need beta blockers)
Hypertension: (may need nitroglycerin and/or nitroprusside)
Mobitz type II
3° AV Block (may require a pacemaker)
Left Bundle Branch Block
Right Bundle Branch Block
Cardiogenic Shock

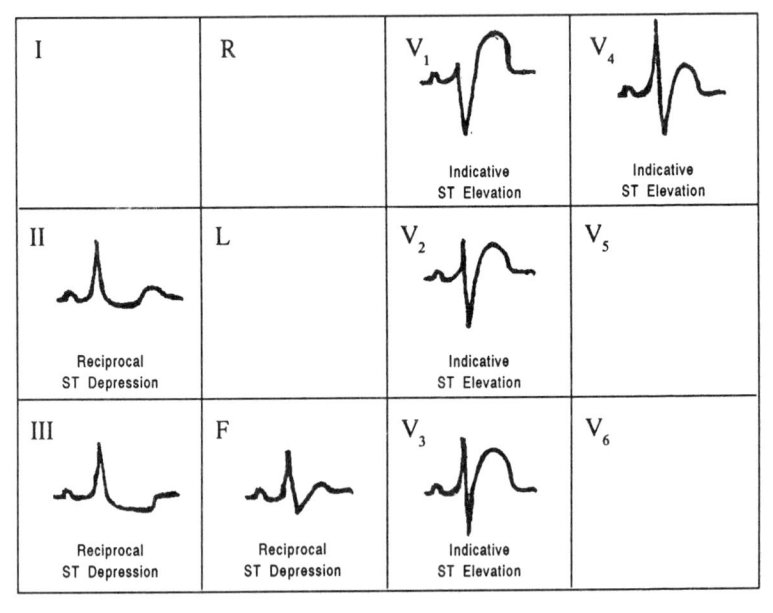

I	R	V_1 Indicative ST Elevation	V_4 Indicative ST Elevation
II Reciprocal ST Depression	L	V_2 Indicative ST Elevation	V_5
III Reciprocal ST Depression	F Reciprocal ST Depression	V_3 Indicative ST Elevation	V_6

SEPTAL MI

Indicative Leads: Loss of R wave in V_1 and/or V_2 and V_3

Reciprocal Leads: None

Arterial Perfusion: The Left Anterior Descending Artery supplies most of the ventricular septum. Septal Perforating Arteries of the LAD perfuse the anterior and inferior septum.

The Posterior Descending Artery (which is usually derived from the Right Coronary Artery but is sometimes derived from the Left Circumflex Artery) supplies the superior posterior portion of the ventricular septum.

Potential Complications: Ventricular Septal Defect (VSD)

I	R	V_1 Loss of R wave	V_4
II	L	V_2 Loss of R wave	V_5
III	F	V_3 Loss of R wave	V_6

LATERAL WALL MI

Indicative Leads: I, aVL, V_5 - V_6

Reciprocal Lead: V_1 (sometimes)

Arterial Perfusion: Circumflex Artery

Potential Complications: Conduction defects are rarely seen

Infarctions of the lateral wall usually occur as a result of extension of anterior or inferior wall MIs.

I Indicative ST Elevation	R	V_1 Reciprocal ST Depression	V_4
II	L Indicative ST Elevation	V_2	V_5 Indicative ST Elevation
III	F	V_3	V_6 Indicative ST Elevation

INFERIOR WALL MI

Indicative Leads: II, III, aVF

Reciprocal Leads: 1, aVL

Arterial Perfusion: Right Coronary Artery

Potential
Complications: Parasympathetic Hyperactivity
　　　　　　　　　Bradycardia (may need atropine)
　　　　　　　　　Hypotension
　　　　　　　　　1° AV Block — usually transient
　　　　　　　　　Accelerated Idioventricular Rhythm —
　　　　　　　　　　a response to hypodynamic circulation

I Reciprocal ST Depression	R	V_1	V_4
II Indicative ST Elevation	L Reciprocal ST Depression	V_2	V_5
III Indicative ST Elevation	F Indicative ST Elevation	V_3	V_6

POSTERIOR WALL MI

Indicative Leads: None on anterior chest wall

Reciprocal Leads: V_1 and V_2

Arterial Perfusion: Posterior Descending Artery — usually arises from the Right Coronary Artery but can arise from the Circumflex Artery.

Potential Complications: Posterior Wall MIs can occur as isolated events or in conjunction with Inferior and Lateral Wall MIs. Because of the large amount of posterior wall damage Ventricular irritability is common early.

* *Suspect a posterior infarct when tall R waves are present in V1 or V2 especially when they are accompanied by ST depression in these leads. You can apply the famous "mirror test:" Flip over the EKG, turn it upside down and hold it up to the light. Now the tall R waves are deep Q waves and ST depression becomes ST elevation.*

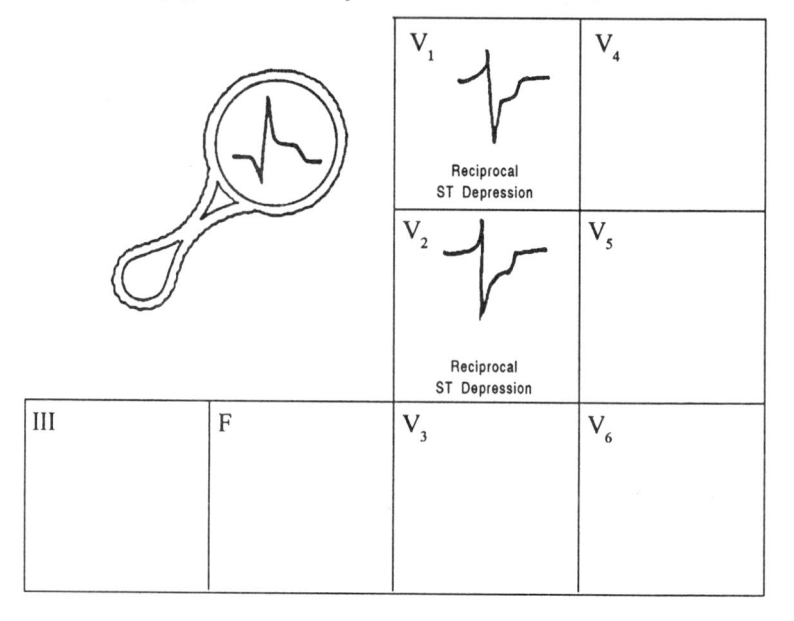

		V_1 Reciprocal ST Depression	V_4
		V_2 Reciprocal ST Depression	V_5
III	F	V_3	V_6

RIGHT VENTRICULAR MI

Indicative Leads: V_2R, V_3R and especially V_4R

Reciprocal Leads: V_1R and possibly V_2R

If you see - on a standard left-sided EKG — ST elevation in V_1 — especially if it is accompanied by ST depression in V_2 — do a right-sided EKG. Then you will see ST depression in V_1R with ST elevation in V_2R, V_3R, and V_4R

Arterial Perfusion: Right Coronary Artery

Potential Complications: AV Block
Hypotension
Shock

Right Ventricular MI on a Right-sided EKG

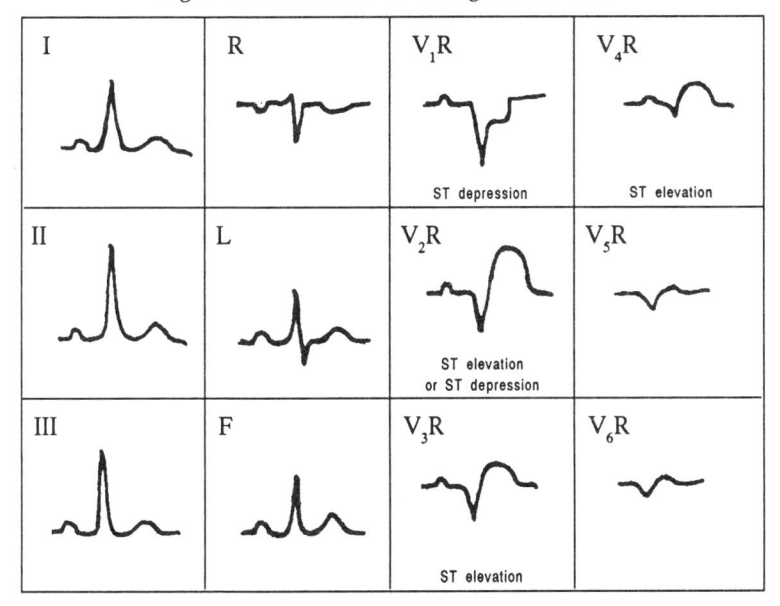

I	R	V_1R ST depression	V_4R ST elevation
II	L	V_2R ST elevation or ST depression	V_5R
III	F	V_3R ST elevation	V_6R

PERRY CARDITIS

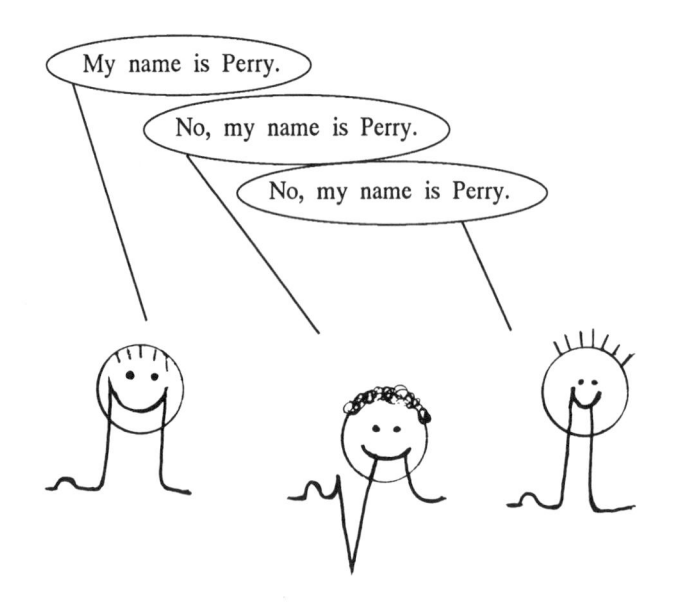

My name is Perry.

No, my name is Perry.

No, my name is Perry.

To tell the truth – we're all Perry.

Perry Happy

Perry Smiley

Perry Global

PERICARDITIS

"I HAVE CHEST PAIN. It's sharp and stab-stab-stabbing me and I can feel it in my back and neck. I hurt and I'm uptight," says the tall worried man in a skimpy blue and white polka-dotted hospital gown.

When you auscultate his chest you hear the sound of footsteps crunching in snow and recognize it as a pericardial friction rub. After you call for a stat EKG, you ask him a few questions. You're concerned because pericarditis would predispose this man to atrial tachyarrythmias, especially if he has an underlying condition such as coronary artery disease or cardiomyopathy.

"Yes," he answers you. "it does hurt more when I take a deep breath and I do feel better sitting up and leaning forward."

The EKG taken shows it clearly — classic Stage 1 pericarditis. EKGs don't always shows pericarditis but this one does. Global "smiling" ST segments, no reciprocal changes. You look at his EKGs from last week. the Q waves are from the MI he had five days ago; there are no new ones.

A normal variant, early repolarization, can mimic the pattern of pericarditis but this you would expect from a healthy individual with no chest pain. The patient history is always the most important element in the big picture.

STAGES OF PERICARDITIS

The stages of acute pericarditis are variable but each one usually last ten days to two weeks.

Stage 1, the ST Stage: There is diffuse "smiley" ST elevation in all the leads except aVR, aVL, III and V_1. In leads aVL, III and V_1 the ST segment may be isoelectric, depressed, or elevated. In aVR the ST segment will be depressed.

Usually there are no coved ST segments and no reciprocal changes. The ventricular subepicardium experiences a general involvement with the irritation of the pericardium — most of the time. Occasionally there will be a localized involvement of the subepicardium with smiley ST elevation restricted to a few leads and with reciprocal ST depression. But for the most part *ST elevation is global and there are no reciprocal changes.* You should not see new Q waves. The T waves are upright.

The PR interval is often displaced, probably representing atrial involvement. Do not use the PR interval to identify the baseline when you suspect pericarditis. Use the TP segment instead.

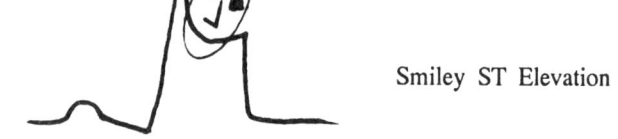

Stage 1   Smiley ST Elevation

Stage 2, Pseudonomalization: This stage can be deceptive — it can look so normal. T waves are upright. The ST segment is isoelectric. It is interesting to note that T waves are upright in stage 1 and stage 2 of pericarditis — in sharp contrast to the inverted T waves of acute MI. The PR interval may or may not be depressed.

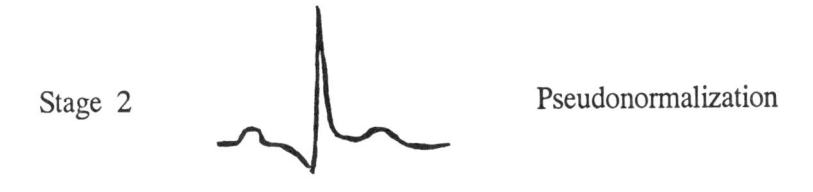

Stage 2   Pseudonormalization

Stage 3, the T Stage: Now you will see diffuse T wave inversion in the leads that had smiley ST segment elevation. The ST segment now is isoelectric.

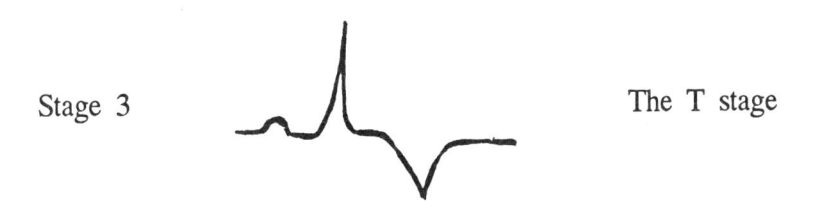

Stage 3   The T stage

State 4, Resolution: In stage 4 the complex resumes its former shape.

PERICARDITIS

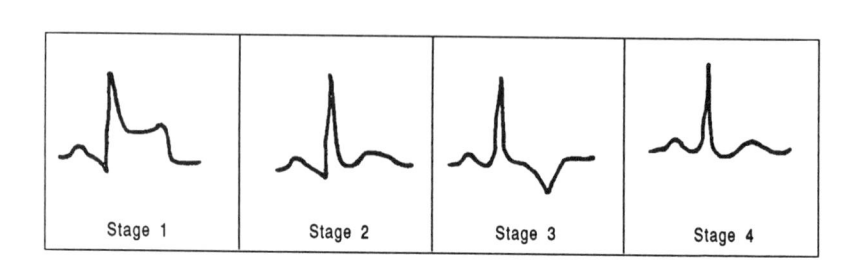

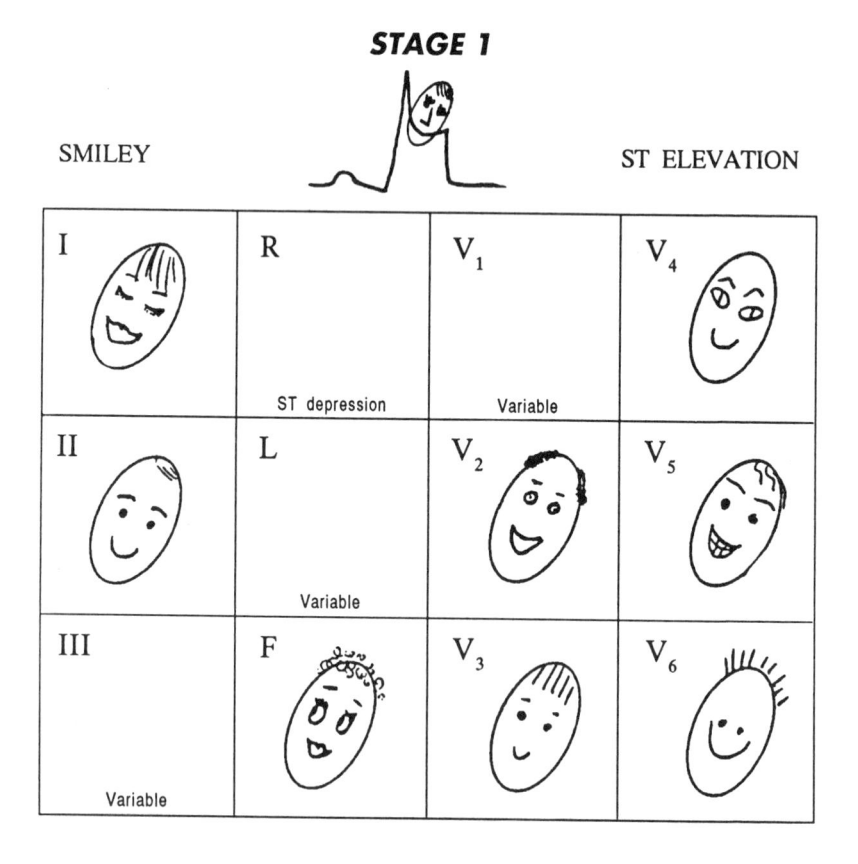

Stage 1	Stage 2	Stage 3	Stage 4

STAGE 1

SMILEY   ST ELEVATION

I	R	V_1	V_4
	ST depression	Variable	
II	L	V_2	V_5
	Variable		
III	F	V_3	V_6
Variable			

SECTION THREE

HYPERTROPHY, BUNDLE BRANCH BLOCK, AND ECTOPY

I must say, as a group we love games. Tug-of-war is a particular favorite.

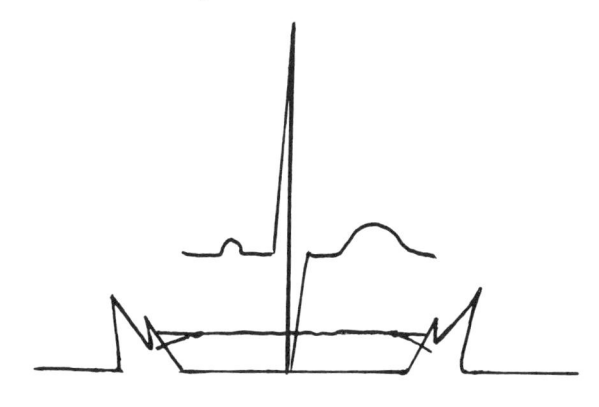

The Fairytale Continues . . .

Like Reading a Snowflake

Dr. Finebeat was satisfied with Princess Infarction's progress. She had responded beautifully to rotor-rooter-ase, her ST segments were back to baseline — only a Q wave in the V_1 - V_3 leads stood testimony to her anterior infarction. She was doing so well, in fact, that Dr. Finebeat had sent her to begin cardiac rehab last month.

How was he to know that cardiac rehab was run by the mad scientist wearing a clever disguise?

If only Prince Ischemia thought his care was going so well. The unhappy royal had ordered a number of EKG books and studied them diligently. Two weeks ago he stormed into the office claiming to be having a non-Q wave MI. When the lab techs reported no abnormal elevation in his cardiac enzymes, Prince Ischemia went to the lab and demanded to be shown the process of spinning the results. An exhausted staff finally left the lab at midnight.

Next the Prince decided he had a posterior wall MI. He came to the office raving, "Mirror, mirror on the posterior wall, who is the most neglected of them all?"

Again the EKG and enzymes were negative. When the Prince found out about the negative results, he returned to the lab and terrorized the crew. Now the Prince carries a mirror with him wherever he goes.

Today, he had come to the office convinced he was having an infarction masked by a left bundle branch block. Today the lab technicians — all of them in Dr. Finebeat's favorite lab — had quit their jobs.

Much as Dr. Finebeat liked working with Zephanie Zucker, he felt she added to the problem — all this patient advocate stuff. **What about being my advocate?** he brooded.

Zephanie had actually once mentioned to the Prince that interpretation of EKGs was a complex thing, that one problem can conceal another — that reading an EKG is like reading a snowflake! What had she said? Each is individual, unique, the fingerprint of forces we are just beginning to truly understand." These days Prince Ischemia wears a platinum snowflake on all his lapels.

Today Prince Ischemia told Dr. Finebeat his "cardiac fingerprints" were melting with the heat of the EKG stylus. Zephanie was teaching him all these words! At least she had the grace to blush with the fingerprint-snowflake reference. But of course she had to go on and ruin it by suggesting that the Prince be taught to do his own EKGs, to own and operate his own machine for a greater sense of security. She was working out a way for him to do this, practicing with him right now. They were both snowflakes in Dr. Finebeat's opinion. But hey, if it keeps him out of my office, thought the doctor, it's wonderful, wonderful, wonderful with me.

Needless to say the same thought had crossed Zephanie's mind, too. But she was beginning to experience a chilly doubt that that would ever happen. Poor Prince Ischemia stood before her at this very moment, clutching a perfectly normal sinus rhythm EKG in his hand. His eyes were frantic. He cried, "I know I have a left bundle branch block — maybe it's rate-related. Please, just one more EKG?"

HYPERTROPHY, BUNDLE BRANCH BLOCK AND ECTOPY

COGNITIVE OBJECTIVES

* Identify the characteristics of left ventricular hypertrophy according to the Cornell criteria.

* Describe the changes seen in right and left atrial abnormalities.

* Identify right and left bundle branch blocks.

* Identify anterior and posterior hemiblocks.

* Describe the arterial perfusion of the left anterior and posterior fasicles.

* Describe how to diagnose myocardial infarction in the presence of a left bundle branch block.

* Identify ST-T changes seen in bundle branch blocks

* Define the term, aberration.

* Identify the shapes of complexes associated with SVT with aberration and with ventricular ectopy.

CHAMBER ENLARGEMENT AND HYPERTROPHY

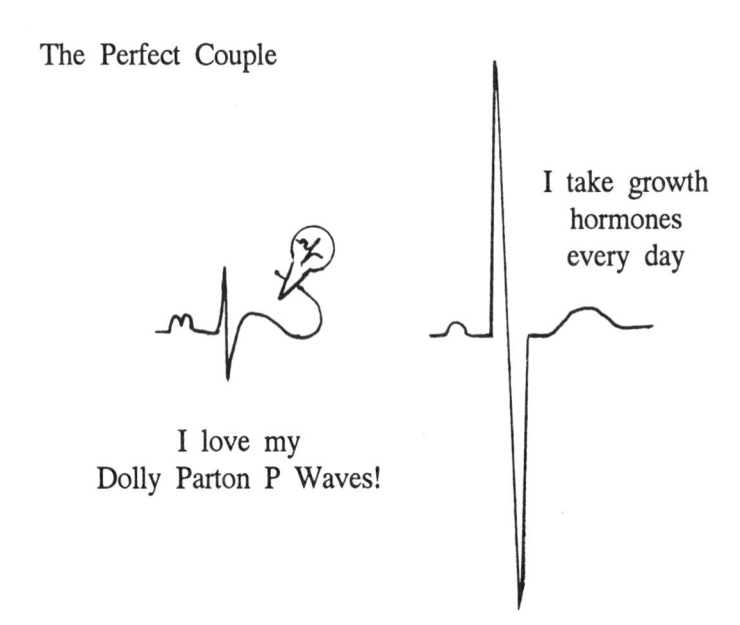

The Perfect Couple

I take growth hormones every day

I love my Dolly Parton P Waves!

We work hard at being the perfect couple.

CHAMBER ENLARGEMENT AND HYPERTROPHY

The echocardiogram is fast replacing the EKG as the tool for detecting chamber enlargement. It's no wonder why. Patients with chamber enlargement and hypertrophy can have normal-looking EKGs. Maybe they're obese or have COPD. Air and fat don't conduct electricity well. Or — our favorite — maybe its a normal variant. On the other hand, people with normal hearts can meet the criteria for chamber enlargement and/or hypertrophy. Maybe they have chests with thin walls — or maybe it's just a normal variant.

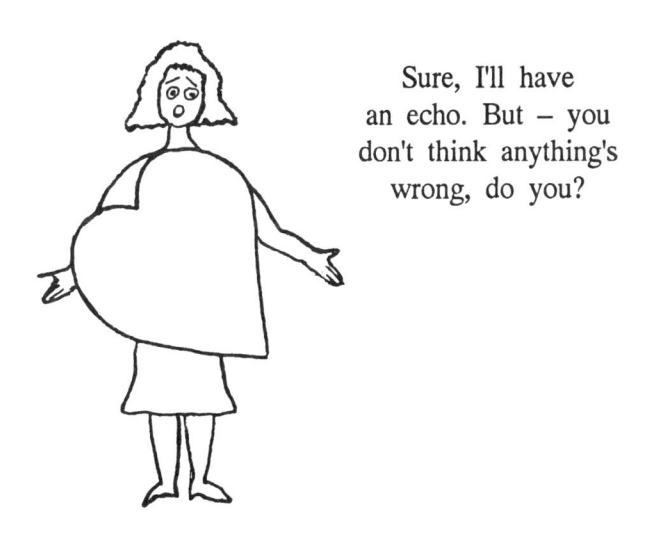

Sure, I'll have an echo. But – you don't think anything's wrong, do you?

Probably you want to know the criteria anyway ...

ATRIAL ABNORMALITIES

A normal P wave does not exceed 2.5 millimeters in height or 0.11 seconds in duration. It has a nice round shape, flattened a little at the top.

The right atrium kicks off depolarization from the sinus node and the electrical activity of the *right* atrium forms the *beginning* shape of the P wave while the depolarization of the *left* atrium forms the *tail* of the P wave. When the right atrium becomes enlarged, the P wave becomes tall and peaked but not wide.

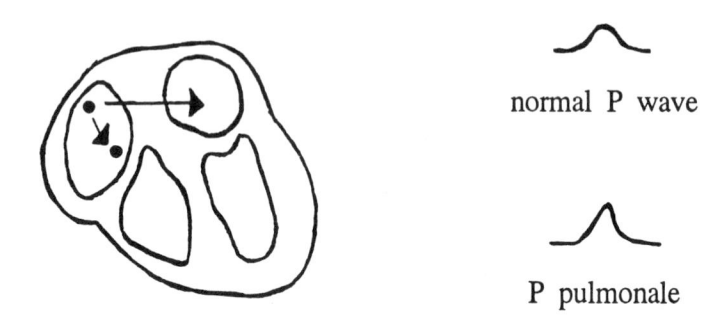

normal P wave

P pulmonale

To qualify the *right atrial abnormality* (RAA), the P wave must reach or exceed 2.6 mm in one of the inferior leads II, III or aVF. A tall peaked P wave is called "P pulmonale" because it often keeps company with pulmonary conditions such as pulmonary stenosis or chronic obstructive pulmonary disease.

Left atrial abnormality (LAA) is determined by the second half of the P wave. Increased *width* of 0.12 seconds or more, often with a notched appearance, is suggestive of LAA. Slight notching can be normal but a peak-to-peak interval of 0.04 seconds (one baby box) or greater is indicative of LAA. Finally, a look at lead V1 is in order. If the "terminal deflection" of the P wave is one baby box deep and one baby box wide, think LAA.

Notched P waves are often called "P mitrale" because they have been associated with mitral stenosis. They are also associated with left and right atrial enlargement, left ventricular hypertrophy and impaired left ventricular function, and coronary artery disease.

Dolly Parton P waves in Lead II

Is the terminal deflection one box wide and one box deep in V_1?

Right and left atrial abnormality used to be called right and left enlargement (RAE and LAE) but the term *abnormality* is preferred now because it is more general.

VENTRICULAR HYPERTROPHY

Pressure or volume overload cause hypertrophy and chamber enlargement. Often the two go hand in hand. For instance, a valvular insufficiency causing a back flow of blood into a ventricle will enlarge the chamber while its walls will thicken to accommodate the weight.

Causes of *left ventricular hypertrophy* include systemic hypertension, aortic stenosis, aortic insufficiency, coarctation of the aorta and hypertrophic cardiomyopathy.

Causes of *right ventricular hypertrophy* include both mitral and tricuspid insufficiency, pulmonic hypertension and chronic lung diseases, and congenital lesions such as the tetralogy of Fallot, pulmonic stenosis and transposition of the great vessels.

Left Ventricular Hypertrophy

The walls of the left ventricle in the *normal* adult heart are about three times as thick as the walls of the right ventricle. When the left ventricle squeezes its blood into all our burger king arteries, it generates up to ten times the force of the right ventricle squirting its blood to the lungs. So, of course the QRS we see on the EKG is a picture of the left ventricle doing its impressive thing.

Normal Heart

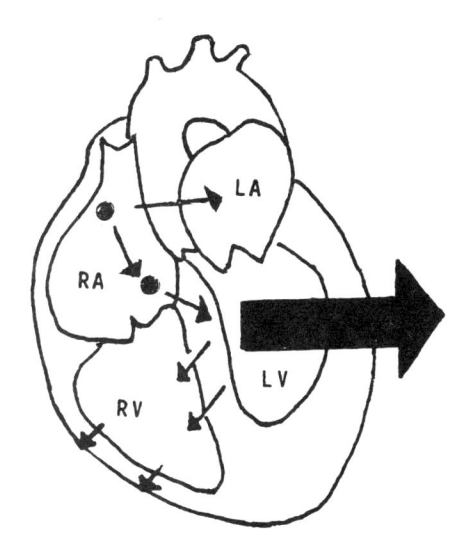

Left ventricle's walls 3x as thick as right ventricle's.

Force of ejection up to 10x as great

So what happens when the powerful left ventricle enlarges? The QRS gets bigger.

One of the simplest criteria for left ventricular hypertrophy is the *"Cornell voltage."* This formula has a *sensitivity* of 42% (sensitivity refers to the recognition of a condition) and a *specificity* of 96% (specificity means the diagnosis confirmed by another test, such as catherization, echo or autopsy). It's accuracy is fairly good and it's very simple:

CORNELL VOLTAGE CRITERION FOR LVH

Add the height of the R wave in aVL
+ the depth of the S wave in V3 =

If the sum equals more than 28 mm in men or 20 mm in women, LVH is present

Be aware that many EKG machines scale precordial leads to one-half size when high-amplitude QRS complexes are registered and this scaling will be noted on the tracing.

Strain

Strain often accompanies ventricular hypertrophy. The reasons for strain are not clear but it is believed that conduction delays through the thickened walls and ischemia due to an increase in the diameter of the muscle fibers play an important role.

Left Ventricular Strain

Left ventricular strain is manifested in the EKG by ST depression with asymmetric T wave inversion in leads that face the left ventricle: 1, aVL, V_5 and V_6. Reciprocal ST elevation with upright T waves are seen in leads that face the right ventricle: V_1 and V_2.

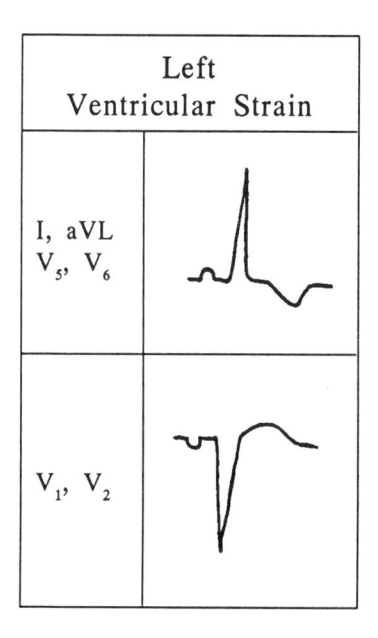

Left Ventricular Strain	
I, aVL V$_5$, V$_6$	
V$_1$, V$_2$	

Right Ventricular Hypertrophy

For right ventricular hypertrophy to show itself on an EKG, it has to be very, very, very bad. After all, the activities of the left ventricle usually control the stylus of the EKG machine.

There are three kinds of right ventricular hypertrophy. Lead V$_1$ is a good clue to what's happening since it faces the right ventricle.

Type A RVH: V₁ shows a large R wave. Type A occurs in congenital heart diseases such as pulmonary stenosis, tetralogy of Fallot, and Eisenmenger's syndrome.

Type B RVH: V₁ shows an equiphasic complex. Congenital conditions can cause this type of right ventricular hypertrophy although type B is less severe than Type A. Additional causes include mitral stenosis, pulmonary hypertension and cor pulmonale.

Type C RVH: V₁ shows an rSr′ or rSR′ pattern. Poor wave progression is seen across the V leads while S waves stubbornly persist. Low voltage in the limb leads is frequently seen. Type C RVH is common in adults, often caused by pulmonary disease.

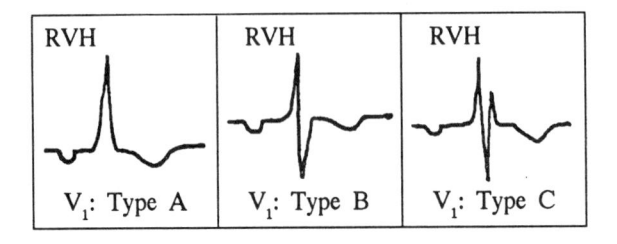

RVH	RVH	RVH
V₁: Type A	V₁: Type B	V₁: Type C

Criterion For RVH

Right axis deviation

R:S ratio in V_1 greater than 1.0

R wave in V_1 7 mm or more

S wave in V_5 and V_6 equal to 7 mm

R wave in V_1 + S wave in V_5 or V_6 greater than 10 mm

rSr' in V_1 with R' greater than 10 mm
q R or qRS pattern in V_1

Right ventricular strain pattern

Right Ventricular Strain

Right ventricular strain will show the same kind of ST segment changes but in different leads. V_1, V_2, II, III, and aVF will show ST segment depression with asymmetric T wave inversion while V_5 and V_6 will show ST elevation with upright T waves.

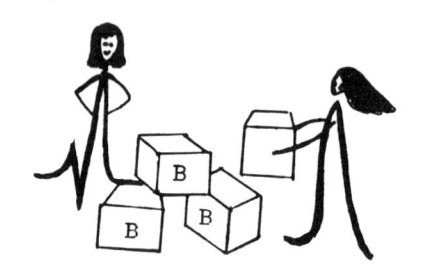

BUNDLE BRANCH BLOCKS

BUNDLE BRANCH BLOCKS

Normally both ventricles are depolarized simultaneously. The left side of the septum receives the impulse first via the left bundle branch. The impulse travels across the thick septum while the right bundle branch catches up. The left side needs a head start because its walls are thicker. The end result is that the ventricles are in perfect step by the time systole comes about. When either the right or left bundle branch is blocked, there is a delay in the conduction pattern and the dance of systole becomes disjointed, conduction wanders — it becomes *aberrant*.

Causes of Bundle Branch Blocks

Occluded arterial perfusion to a bundle branch will cause it to block. Partial occlusion will cause an intermittent block. *Changes in the fibrous skeleton* of the heart can also cause bundle branch blocks. This fibrous skeleton is an intricate structure that houses the muscles and valves of the heart. Congenital deformities, valvular disease and systemic hypertension can affect the fibrous skeleton and thus cause bundle branch blocks.

ARTERIAL PERFUSION OF THE BUNDLE BRANCHES

Right Bundle Branch

The right bundle branch (RBB) is a long slender fiber tract. It begins at the bundle of HIS and threads its way through the interventricular septum to the base of the anterior papillary muscle of the right ventricle. It is supplied with blood by the *AV nodal artery*. The AV nodal artery is found on the back of the heart and springs off the posterior descending artery. Usually the posterior descending artery is fathered by the right coronary artery (RCA) but sometimes it is formed from the left circumflex artery. Additionally in half the population, the right bundle branch is perfused by the *first septal perforator* of the left anterior descending artery (LAD).

Left Bundle Branch

The left bundle branch (LBB) divides into three parts: the left anterior fasicle, the left centroseptal fasicle and the left posterior fasicle.

The **left anterior fasicle** receives its blood from *septal perforating branches* of the LAD and runs from the bundle of HIS to the anterior papillary muscle of the mitral valve.

The **left centroseptal fasicle** can arise from either the anterior or posterior fasicle or from where the fasicles branch apart and it zaps the septum.

The **left posterior fasicle** is a spray of fibers nourished by the *AV nodal artery* and, in some people, by the *septal perforating arteries* of the LAD as well. It finds its way from the bundle of HIS to the posterior papillary muscle of the left ventricle.

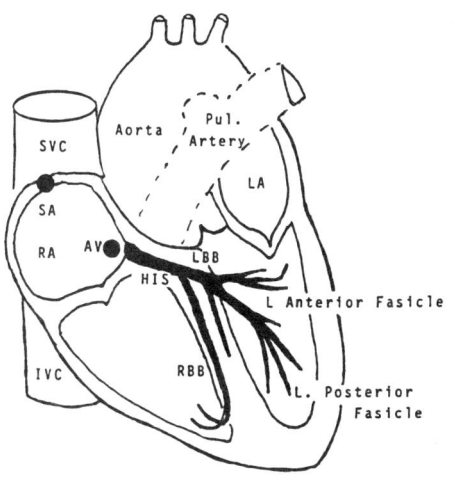

Bundle Branches

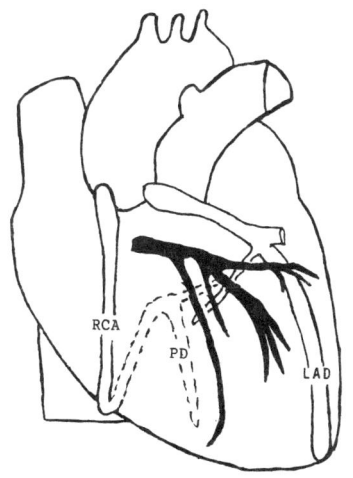

Arterial Perfusion

EKG CHANGES

Right Bundle Branch Block

In right bundle branch block the beginning of the QRS complex is the same as a normal QRS complex because the wave of depolarization starts down its usual path. In V_1 there will be a small R wave as the wave front crosses the septum and in V_6 there will be a small Q wave.

But when the wave of electricity reaches the right bundle, nothing happens. Oh no! Will the right ventricle ever get activated?

The poor wavefront has to go the long way around, wiggling, squiggling, sashaying its way through the muscle — in the "free" walls of the ventricles.

**RBB Out of Order
Take Detour**

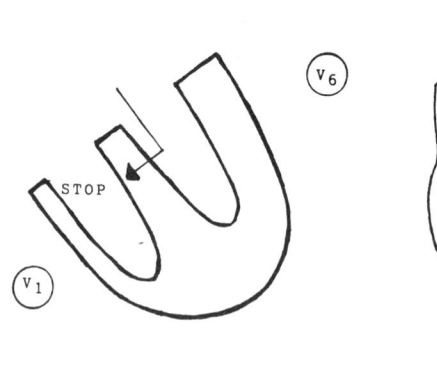

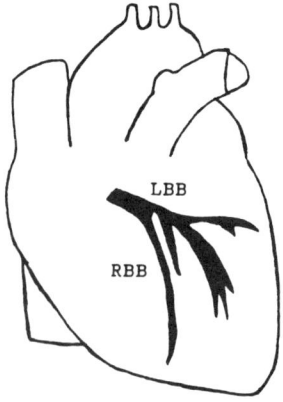

The left ventricle depolarizes on time but the right ventricle lags behind. The right ventricle experiences a "terminal conduction delay" and the ending of the QRS is altered.

In V_1, the lead closest to the right ventricle, look for an rSR´ complex that looks something like this:

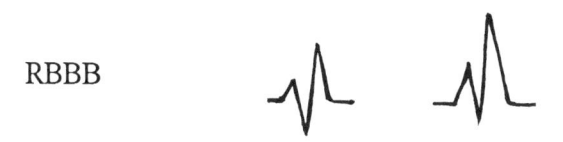

RBBB

Note the famous rabbit ears of a right bundle branch block. Sometimes the R wave will be notched —

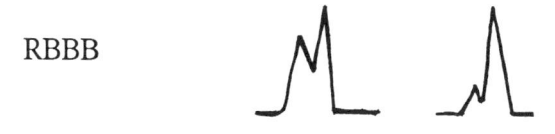

RBBB

Meanwhile in V_6 look for a wide slurred S wave:

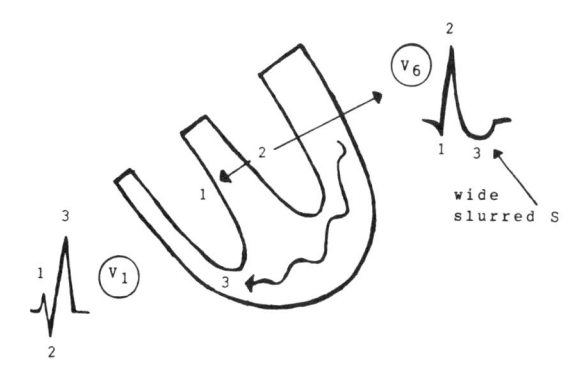

The criteria for a right bundle branch block is a QRS complex that is wider than 0.11 seconds, the presence of an rSR´ complex in V_1 and wide S waves in I, aVL, V_5 and V_6.

It is interesting to note that the pattern of a BBB doesn't mean that the continuity of the branch is disrupted entirely at any given point. What it does mean is that the electrical impulse is travelling faster through the free wall of the other ventricle than through the "blocked" bundle. In fact it may be distant Purkinje fibers of the affected ventricle that are creating the disturbance.

Left Bundle Branch Block

The very beginning of the normal depolarization process is ruined in left bundle branch block. The impulse just can't zip down the left side of the septum.

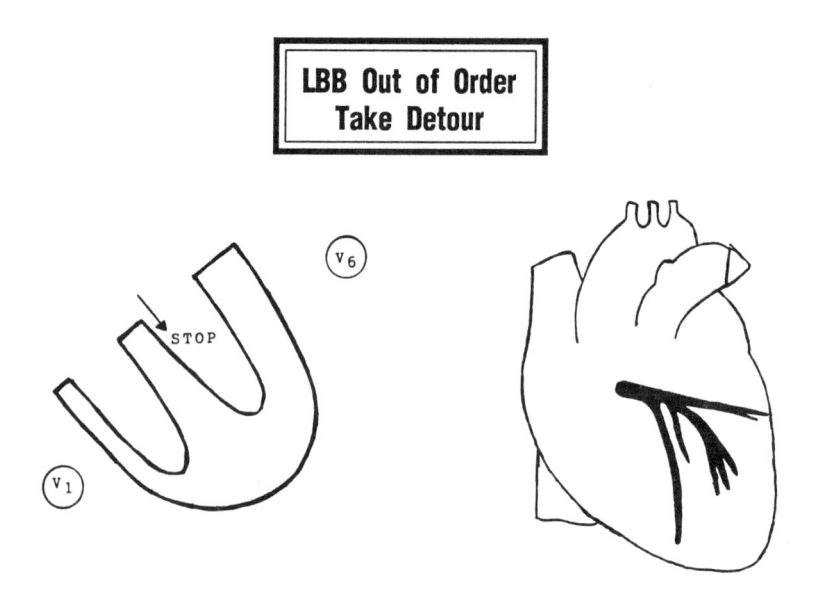

Instead the wavefront accepts its only alternative: it slips down the right bundle branch instead. Then it crosses the septum from *right to left.*

What's the electrocardiographic result? The R wave in V_1 *may* be lost. It may remain if the thin right ventricular free wall becomes activated before the fat septum. V_1, being so close to this right wall *could* pick up the vibes. But *forget* the q wave in V_6; its gone. The R wave in V_6 is usually wide and slurred because the impulse took longer to penetrate the far wall of the left ventricle.

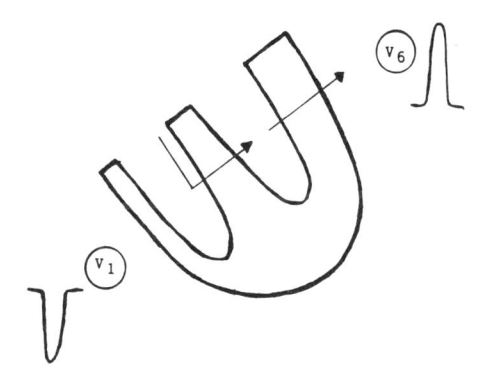

A LBBB can be caused by a block in the main left bundle branch *(predivisional)* or by a block in both the anterior fasicle and the posterior fasicle that occurs simultaneously *(post-divisional).*

The criteria for left bundle branch block is a QRS duration of at least 0.12 seconds, loss of Q waves in I, aVL and V_6 and an R wave in 1, aVL and V_6. This R wave is usually notched or slurred. There is an rS or QS in V_1.

LBBB

Look at	Look for
	QRS of 0.12 secs duration or more
	Late intrinsic deflection (see page 43)
1, aVL, V_6	R waves in 1, aVL and V_6 — usually notched or slurred
	Loss of q waves in I, aVL and V_6
	T waves in opposite direction to terminal portion of QRS
V_1	Negative QRS in V_1

Comparison of RBBB and LBBB in V_1 and V_6

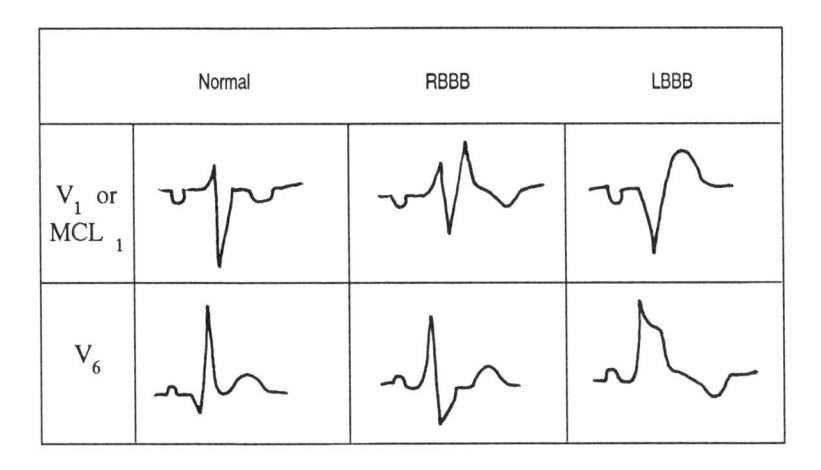

	Normal	RBBB	LBBB
V_1 or MCL$_1$			
V_6			

Please note that in MCL$_1$ (which mimics V_1), an upward deflection denotes right bundle branch block while a negative deflection denotes left bundle branch block — one of the reasons MCL$_1$ is a good lead for constant monitoring.

Incomplete Bundle Branch Block

Incomplete LBBB is diagnosed when the EKG shows a LBBB pattern with a QRS duration of up to 0.12 seconds.

Incomplete RBBB is diagnosed with the EKG shows a RBBB pattern with a QRS duration of up to 0.10 seconds.

Rate-Related Bundle Branch Block

Sometimes BBB develops only when the heart speeds up to a "critical rate." One or the other bundle branch may still be in the refractory period, unable to conduct an impulse. A rate-related BBB develops that will correct itself when the heart rate slows down.

ST-T changes in Bundle Branch Block

The polarity of the ST segment and the T wave in BBB is in opposite direction to the terminal portion of the QRS complex because relaxation of the ventricles is disturbed by the block. Such changes are called *secondary T wave changes* and are considered normal.

If, however, the ST segment and the T wave have the same polarity as the latter portion of the QRS, the heart may be experiencing ischemia as well as the BBB. When this situation happens, it is called a *primary T wave change*.

(Normal) Secondary T Wave Changes		
	RBBB	LBBB
V_1		
V_6		

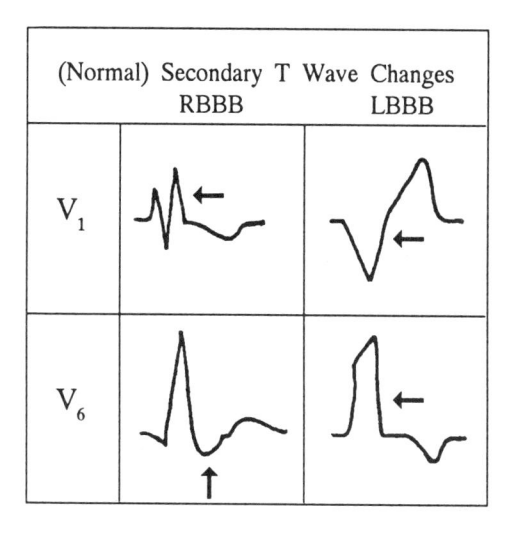

Arrows indicate terminal portions of QRS.
Polarity of ST segments and T waves
is in opposite direction.

RIGHT BUNDLE BRANCH BLOCK (RBBB)

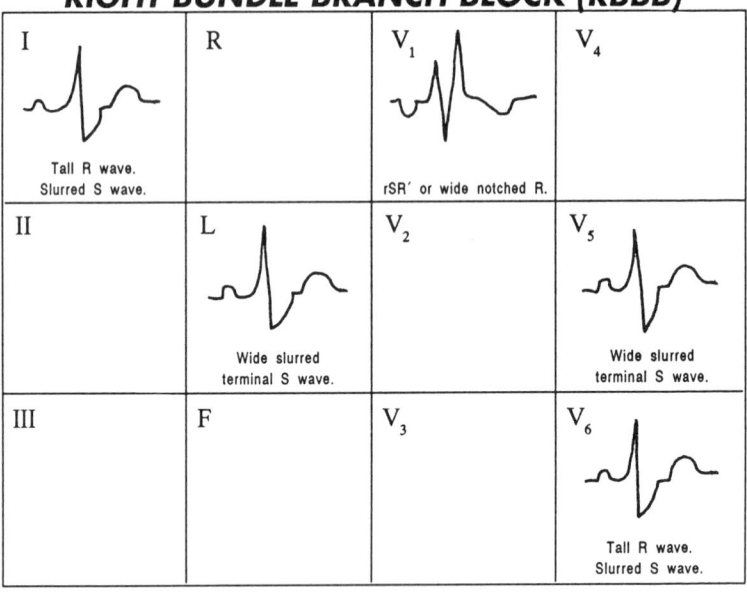

I	R	V₁	V₄
Tall R wave. Slurred S wave.		rSR′ or wide notched R.	
II	L	V₂	V₅
	Wide slurred terminal S wave.		Wide slurred terminal S wave.
III	F	V₃	V₆
			Tall R wave. Slurred S wave.

LEFT BUNDLE BRANCH BLOCK (LBBB)

I	R	V₁	V₄
Notched/slurred R. No Q wave.		rS or QS.	
II	L	V₂	V₅
	Notched/slurred R. No Q wave.		
III	F	V₃	V₆
			Notched/slurred R. No Q wave.

BUNDLE BRANCH BLOCK AND MYOCARDIAL INFARCTION

Right BBB and MI

Right BBB patterns don't contest the patterns of infarction on the EKG and human beings have no problem seeing MI in the midst of RBBB. The initial forces of left to right septal activation are intact so when an MI comes along, Q waves show while ST elevation just superimposes itself on the RBBB pattern. For instance, in V_1 the Q wave and ST elevation of an *anterior septal wall MI* can easily be seen despite the presence of RBBB:

RBBB + MI = RBBB + MI

Lead V_1

If only we could say the same about LBBB!

Left BBB and MI

Left bundle branch block definitely interferes with the diagnosis of MI. Septal activation in LBBB is reversed and goes from right to left, thanks to the intact right bundle branch. Left bundle branch block, with its potent right to left energy, can squash the Q waves of anterior and interior infarctions. To add insult to injury (so to speak) LBBB in the right precordial leads displays a QS complex with secondary ST-T changes. Look at V_1 now with an *anterior septal wall MI* and LBBB:

LBBB + MI = LBBB + MI

= WHAT?

So what do we search for?

One thing to look for in V_1 and V_2 is a disproportional elevation of the ST segment to more than 8 mm or one half the height of the T wave:

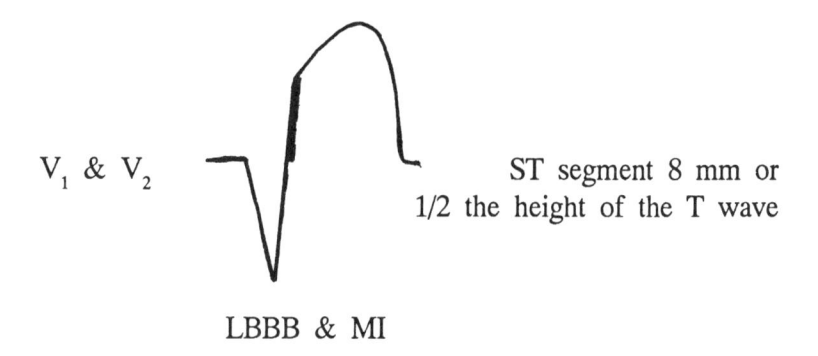

V_1 & V_2 ST segment 8 mm or
                      1/2 the height of the T wave

LBBB & MI

With LBBB even a simple upright T wave in V_5 or V_6 is suspicious. It shows a primary T wave change where you expect to see a secondary T wave change. In any lead a primary ST or T wave change bears investigation. ANYTHING TO DRIVE YOU CRAZY!

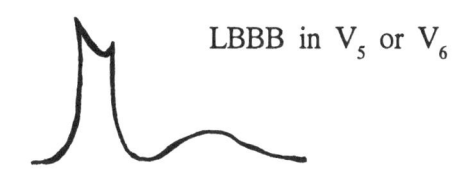

LBBB in V_5 or V_6

Primary T wave change indicative of ischemia

Q Waves

Q waves in LBBB in leads I, V_5 or V_6 — that are 0.04 seconds or longer in duration — shout out MI. These Q waves may reveal the depolarization of the right ventricle or the deflection of current away from dead tissue. In any case, they are abnormal and indicate *anteroseptal or lateral infarction.*

Another finding mentioned by some authors is the presence of funny w-shaped Q waves in leads II, III, and aVF that suggest an *inferior wall infarct.*

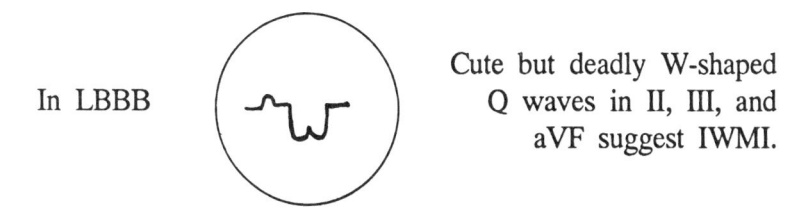

In LBBB

Cute but deadly W-shaped Q waves in II, III, and aVF suggest IWMI.

A. LBBB + Anteroseptal MI

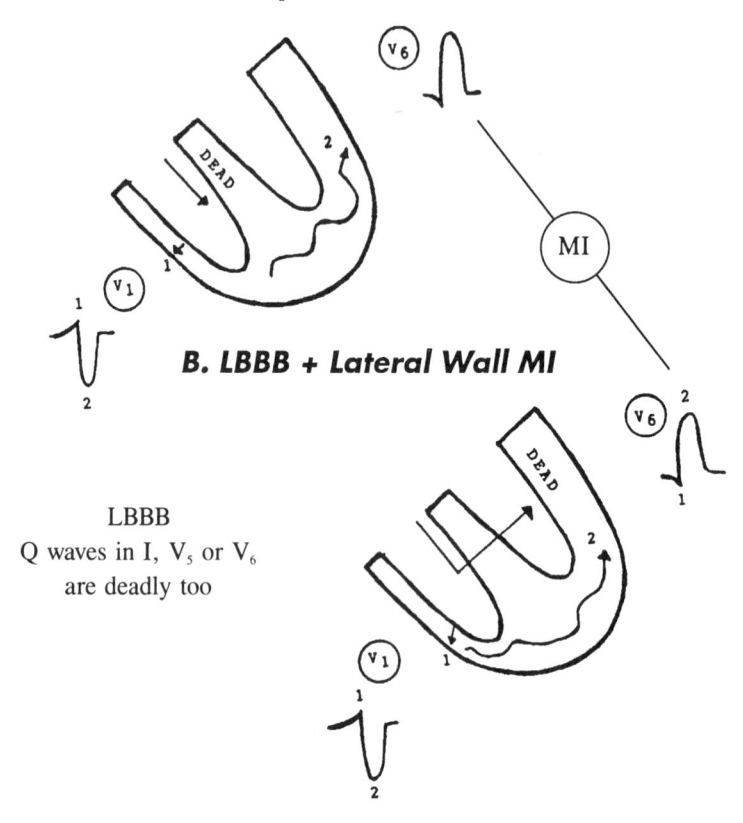

B. LBBB + Lateral Wall MI

LBBB
Q waves in I, V_5 or V_6
are deadly too

Q Waves in V_6 may reveal depolarization of the right ventricle and loss of the septum (A) or deflection of electrical impulse away from dead tissue in lateral wall (B).

Despite the best efforts of the most talented EKG detective in the world, myocardial infarction can stay lost in the shadows of left bundle branch block — forever.

HEMIBLOCKS

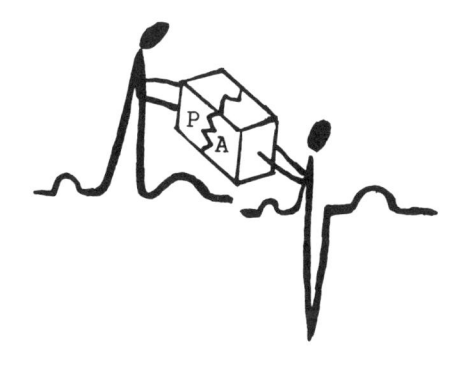

HEMIBLOCKS

Hemiblock is a left-sided block that happens when either the left anterior fasicle or the left posterior fasicle doesn't depolarize its territory. Attempts to correlate EKG patterns of hemiblock with appropriate lesions postmortem have been mostly unsuccessful. This may be because the anterior and posterior fasicles of the left bundle are not truly separate and distinct entities but are a multitude of conduction fibers than run in two basic directions and that enjoy many connections between them.

Left Anterior Hemiblock (LAH)

Left anterior hemiblock, also called *left anterior fasicular block (LAFB),* is quite common. It's only blood supply is the first septal perforator of the LAD. When the *anterior* fasicle is blocked, the *posterior* fasicle depolarizes the left ventricle. This changes the normal direction of depolarization into a left axis deviation. Usually it takes only slightly longer to depolarize via one fasicle (about 0.02 seconds longer) and so the duration of the QRS is usually within normal limits.

The criteria for LAH is based on the features of left axis deviation: *a qR complex in lead I and aVL* with small Q waves and tall R waves and *an RS complex in II, III, and aVF* (left axis deviation) with a small R wave and deep terminal S wave. Often a terminal R wave in aVR is seen as well as increased QRS voltage in the limb leads.

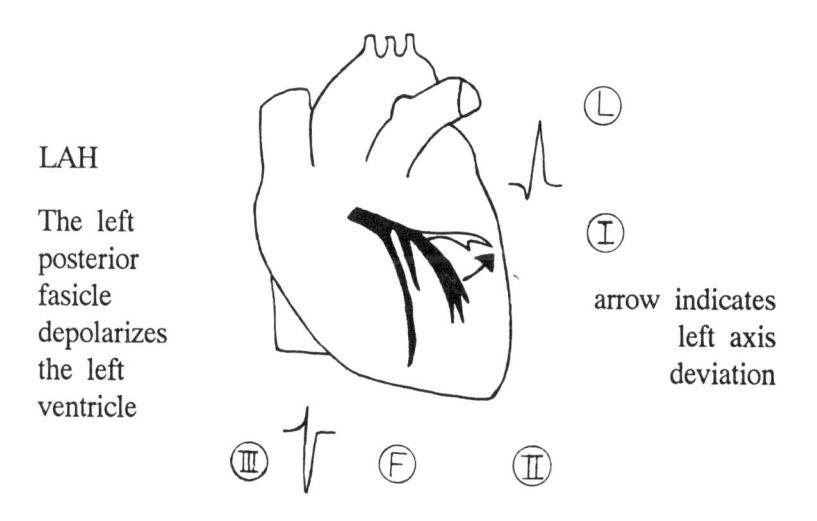

LAH

The left posterior fasicle depolarizes the left ventricle

arrow indicates left axis deviation

LAH often occurs with right bundle branch block. When this happens, it's called a *bifasicular block.*

Left Posterior Hemiblock (LPH)

Also called *left posterior fasicular block (LPFB)*, left posterior hemiblock rarely occurs without concurrent right bundle branch block. Even when it is associated with RBBB, LAH is an oddity. A short thick fasicle that enjoys a dual blood supply from the anterior and posterior arteries, the posterior fasicle is positioned in the left ventricle out of the way of turbulence. It lives the good life.

In the presence of LPH, the left ventricle is depolarized by the anterior fasicle and so right axis deviation is the foundation of the criteria for this block.

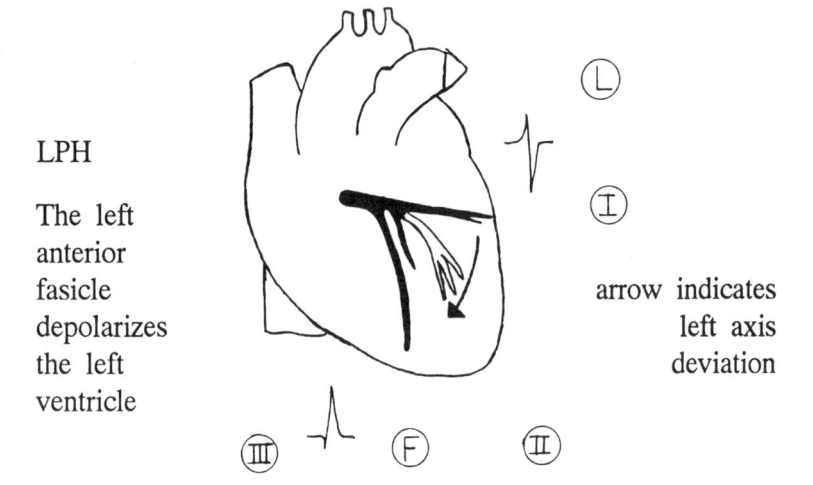

LPH

The left anterior fasicle depolarizes the left ventricle

arrow indicates left axis deviation

Right axis deviation can be caused by other things such as right ventricular hypertrophy, lateral wall infarction, chronic obstructive pulmonary disease and a normal vertical heart. Such conditions should be ruled out before LPH is ruled in.

The criterion for LPH is an *rS complex in leads I and aVL* (right axis deviation) with a small r wave and a deep S wave and a *qR complex in leads II, III, and aVF* with a small Q wave and a tall R wave. The QRS interval can be normal or slightly prolonged. When LPH occurs with RBBB, the QRS can be up to 0.12 seconds.

LEFT ANTERIOR HEMIBLOCK (LAH)

I Small Q wave. Tall R wave.	R	V_1	V_4
II Left Axis Deviation. Small R wave. Deep S wave.	L Small Q wave. Tall R wave.	V_2	V_5
III Left Axis Deviation. Small R wave. Terminal S wave.	F Left Axis Deviation. Small R wave. Deep S wave.	V_3	V_6

LEFT POSTERIOR HEMIBLOCK (LPH)

I Right Axis Deviation. Small R wave. Deep S wave.	R	V_1	V_4
II Small Q wave. Tall R wave.	L Right Axis Deviation. Small R wave. Deep S wave.	V_2	V_5
III Small Q wave. Tall R wave.	F Small Q wave. Tall R wave.	V_3	V_6

ABERRANCY VERSUS ECTOPY

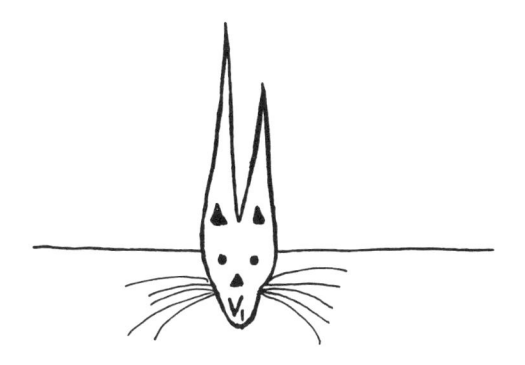

Just what do you mean —
my left ear may mean *trouble?*

ABERRATION

Aberration is ventricular conduction of a supraventricular impulse that is *temporarily* abnormal. One or the other bundle branches is ready to conduct an impulse while the other one isn't. It's like a temporary bundle branch block. Aberration always has an underlying cause and while the cause may be treated, the arrythmia is not.

Runs of supraventricular tachycardia (SVT) with aberrant conduction mimic the shape of ventricular tachycardia (VT) and this is where real problems set in. There are times ventricular ectopy can't be differentiated from SVT with aberrancy but we can reduce confusion substantially by learning to look for a few basic clues.

We can get into healthy habits to help us search. Lead MCL_1 should be used for constant observation of a client. MCL_1 shows off best the contours of right and left bundle branch blocks, aberration and ectopy. Whenever you're in doubt about what you see, check out more than one lead. You can change an MCL_1 to an MCL_6 by switching the positive lead from the 4th intercoastal space at the right sternal border to the 5th intercoastal space at the left anterior axillary line. And by all means, get a twelve-lead EKG.

Aberration is not as frequent as we may think. Henry J.L. Marriott in *Practical Electrocardiography,* says, "Ectopy is much more common than aberration and, when you hear hoofbeats in this Western World, you do not first think of a zebra: you consider the zebra only if you see its stripes." Among his "stripes" of aberration are the following:

Triphasic Contours

Triphasic contours of rsR´ in V_1 and qRs in V_6 are the fingerprints of a right bundle branch block so this morphology speaks in favor of aberration.

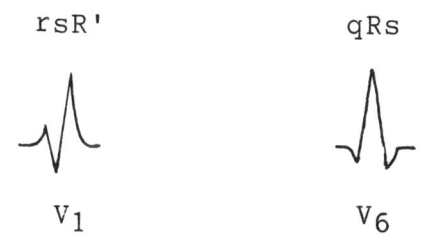

rsR'   qRs

V_1 V_6

Preceding Atrial Activity

When you can find them, P waves before the QRS are great evidence in favor of a supraventricular impulse. P waves are often best seen in the lead with the smallest QRS complex because there you'll find least disturbance of the baseline. Look at all the leads carefully for P waves but if they're not there, don't get hung up on it — go on to other clues.

ALTERNATING BBB PATTERNS

Alternating BBB patterns separated by a single normally conducted beat suggest aberrant conduction. Cardiac care nurses sometimes call this "flipping the bundle."

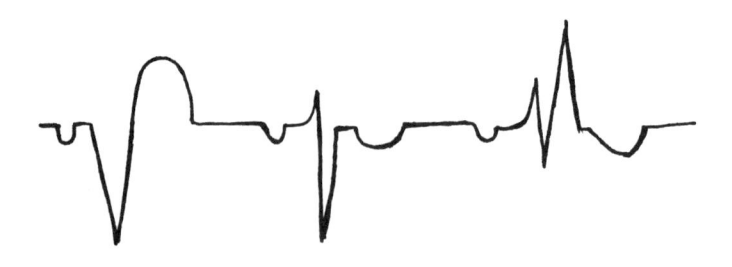

LBBB Pattern					RBBB Pattern

"Flipping the Bundle" in MCL$_1$

PRE-EXISTING BBB

Compare previous tracings when you look at a rhythm you can't identify. If you see a BBB pattern in a conducted rhythm with the same morphology as the rhythm you question, you've lucked into a clue to aberration.

VENTRICULAR ECTOPY

Ventricular ectopy begins with a depolarizing impulse originating in one of the ventricles. The complex is fat and bizarre with no P wave before it.

Right ventricular complexes are negative in V_1. Sometimes the negative complex is preceded by a fat little R wave.

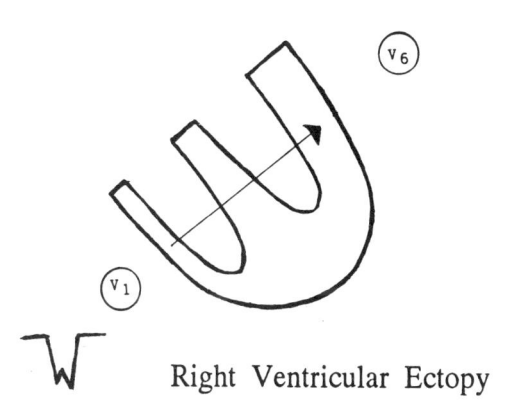

Right Ventricular Ectopy

Left ventricular complexes are positive in V_1 with a monophasic or diphasic shape. Often in the diphasic "rabbit ear" shape, the left rabbit ear will be taller. If the left ear is taller, the weird ugly rhythm you're looking at is probably ventricular ectopy.

Left Ventricular Ectopy

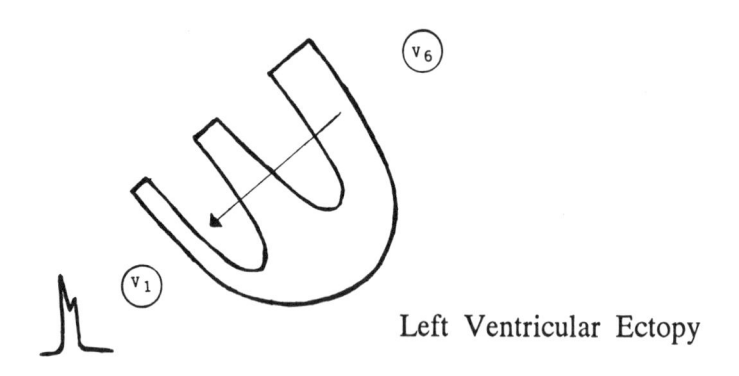

The best way to recognize ventricular ectopy is to memorize its favorite silhouettes against the appearance of aberration. This way you can have a good handle on what's happening most of the time. Please note in the following examples that a contour that denotes aberration in V_1 can denote ectopy in V_6. So you have to know *what shapes in what leads* are dangerous.

Ectopy in V₁   *Aberration in V₁*

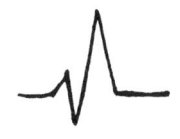

Monophasic R or diphasic qR and rabbit ears with left *or* right ear taller: left ear taller is strong indicator for ectopy.

Triphasic rsR´

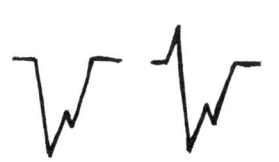

Biphasic rS with fat little R wave

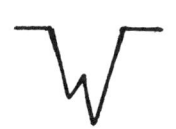

monophasic QS with slurred or notched downstroke

monophasic QS or diphasic rS with slurred or notched upstroke.

Ectopy in V₆   Aberration in V₆

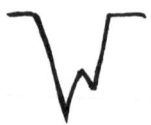

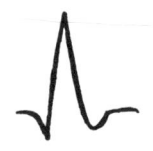

QS with slurred or notched upstroke. Compare this to a similiar shape in V₁

qRs complex with R wave greater than S wave.

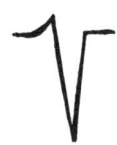

rS with R wave smaller than S wave.

*   *   *

If you see *positive or negative concordance* in the V leads — in which *all* ventricular complexes are either positive or negative, you are probably looking at ventricular ectopy. Another vote for ectopy is an axis in the frontal leads that falls in "No man's land" (a negative complex in Leads I and aVF).

STAMP OUT THE MYTHS

Don't subscribe to the myth that VT is usually irregular whereas SVT is regular. Both VT and SVT can be regular and both VT and SVT can be irregular.

Both VT and SVT can be well tolerated — for hours. Don't be fooled by the client eating breakfast, reading the newspaper with a blood pressure of 120/80 sitting below a monitor that displays a lethal rhythm.

Now would be a good time to ask two very pertinent questions:

"Have you ever had a heart attack?"

"Did the fast beating begin only after the heart attack?"

If the answer to both these questions is yes, you will have gathered a significant piece of evidence in favor of ventricular tachycardia.

A little patient history goes a long way.

	RBBB	LBBB	Rignt Ventricular Ectopy	Left Ventricular Ectopy
V_1 or MCL_1	⅃⋀⌐	⋁	⋁	⋀

AV DISSOCIATION

It's always a good idea to look for clinical signs of AV dissociation when you're deciding if a complex is ventricular or aberrant. Such signs include:

Wide splitting of heart sounds

Variation in the intensity of the first heart sound

Irregular cannon waves in the neck

APPENDIX: DEPOLARIZATION

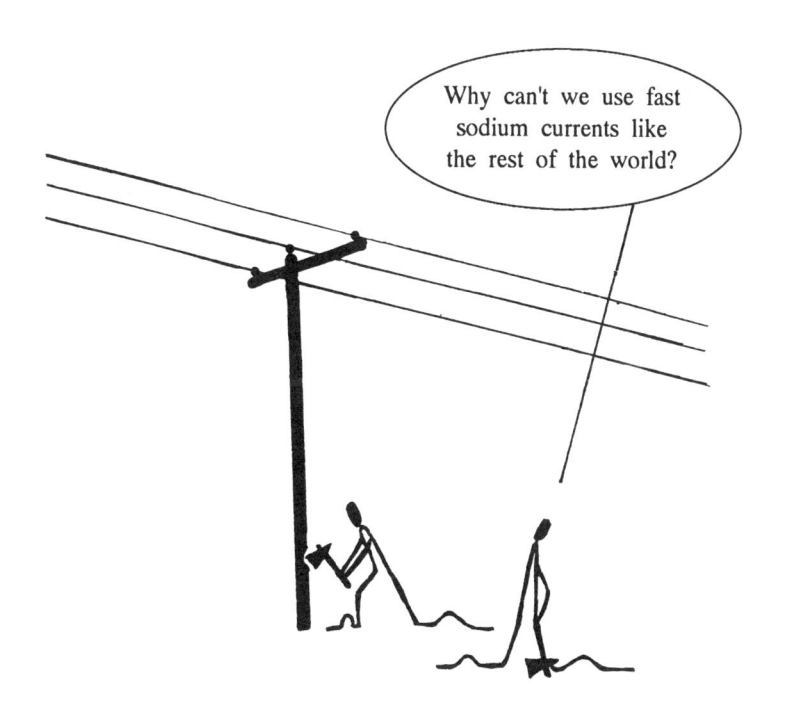

The Fairytale Concludes...

The Reason Behind the Madness

"Do you believe this?" exploded a very exasperated Harrison Potassium the Third. His friends called him HK+3 for short. He was reading a newspaper; you could almost see fumes arising all around his electron shells.

"What, my darling electrolyte?" purred Chlorine Smith, nuzzling up against the irritable element.

Magnesium Calm just watched the two of them. What was it about Potassium that just drew Chlorine to him like a captive slave? All the metals were in love with Chlorine: Magnesium, Sodium, Calcium, and Potassium. *I try the hardest and she goes to all the others before me,* brooded Magnesium. *I am always displaced.*

Chlorine was, in fact, a very fickle amour. Her flirtations caused such trouble that every time Sodium came into a place, Potassium would stalk out through giant protein doors. Humans called it "the sodium-potassium pump." What did they know about true lyte love?

"These earthlings again — they," Harrison Potassium took a deep breath; he was so upset he could hardly speak. "They think there's no life on the moon. What do they call us?"

"That's an old newspaper." Chlorine tried to defuse him.

"*You try to get a more current issue up here!*" Harrison Potassium challenged her. How dare she doubt him and his treasured news-from-the-real world? Had she been with Calcium or worse! with lowly Sodium again?

Usually Magnesium had a sedative effect on things around him but he had had enough for one day. "Harrison Potassium," he fluffed out his electrons a bit. It was awful; he always felt so lightweight around the big K. "I know you like to think we live on our own planet and all — and I realize we are the basic stuff of the universe and exist everywhere and all that. But you and I — we — live in this little cardiac cell in a human on earth."

"His name is Prince Ischemia," added a nearby lipid, doing nothing as usual. Some of us think that you're the reason he's always so neurotic. Maybe these ion consciousness-raising groups that you're organizing in his body are adversely affecting his mind. How's he supposed to be in control? Did you ever think of that?"

"You know, some people say madness is just a chemical thing," chipped in Calcium. "And if the Prince gets too crazy, he could turn into a frog."

"Then we'd really be food for the mad scientist," gasped Peter Protein, who always had something negative to say.

"I heard the mad scientist's running the cardiac rehab lab," said Magnesium. "He doesn't wear a lab coat. He wears dresses and a blue wig. Everyone's fooled by him because he looks so attractive."

Harrison Potassium III

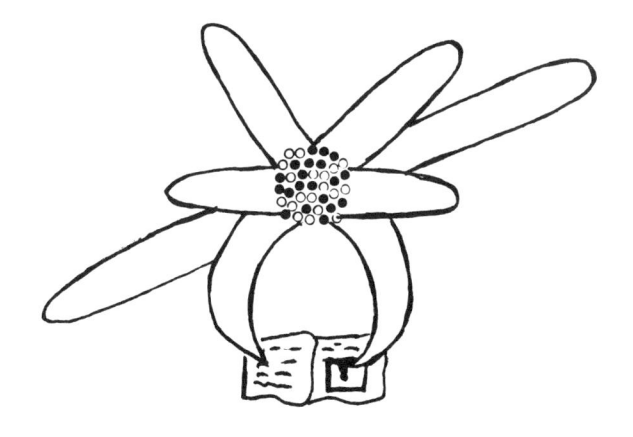

  Harrison Potassium could feel himself to be really on the edge. There was acid-like indigestion in the pit of his nucleus. He just couldn't take much more from these weak beings. Better just to fade out — yes, the darkness is welcome sometimes. Slipping away now. Gone.

CARDIAC CELLS AT REST AND AT WORK

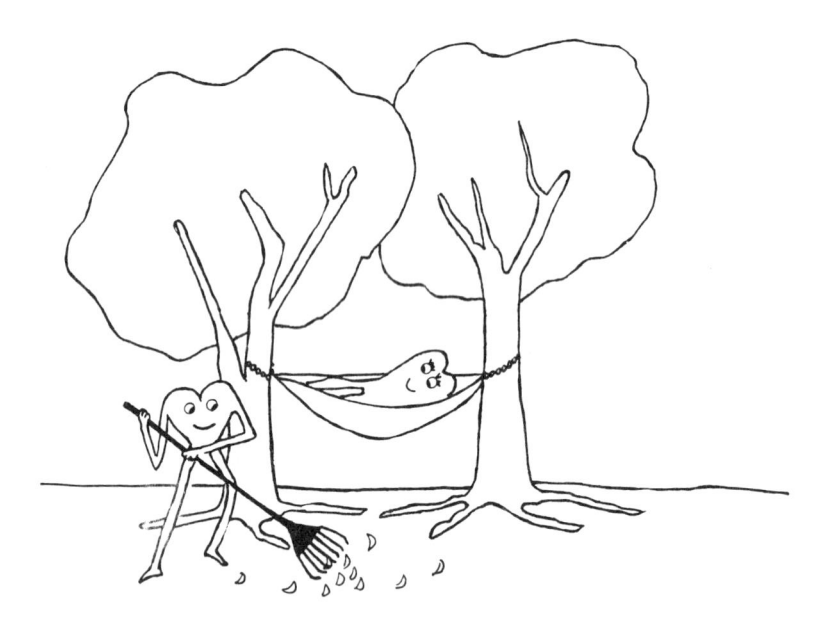

The difference in charge across the cell membrane creates a *"resting membrane potential."* This potential can be thought of as *energy available* due to the *position* of the electrical charges.

The Very Tidy Housekeeping of a Cardiac Muscle Cell

A resting cardiac muscle cell wants every little ion in its proper place because in order for the cell to *relax*, it must maintain a negative charge. *Sodium* must be kept outside. *Calcium* is stored in a network of little tubules called the sarcoplasmic reticulum inside the cell and if calcium is not neatly placed in a tubule, it must leave the cell. As for *potassium,* its place is inside the cell. At times a small amount of potassium is sent outside to adjust the electrical mood of the cell after it contracts.

There are a multitude of mechanisms that assist the cell in maintaining its household. Ongoing research continually reports new findings. Only a few of the well-known phenomenon will be discussed here to provide a very basic overview of how the cell relaxes and how it contracts. *To relax,* the cell must keep its interior negatively charged. To do this it will use passive and active forces.

Passive Forces
Electrochemical Gradients

POTASSIUM. Because there is so much potassium inside the cell and so little outside, a *chemical gradiant* draws potassium out of the cell. But, wait a minute, as too many potassium ions leave the cell, the interior becomes more and more negative and an electrical gradient pulls the positive ions back. Back and forth they go until an *"equilibrium potential"* is reached. The cell wants its inside negative - but not too negative.

Ions move across the cell membrane through protein or phospholipoprotein channels when their "activation gates" are open. The gates may open in response to voltage or substance changes or because of the simple passage of time. Selectivity filters decide which ions can use the channel.

Protein or Phospholipoprotein Channels

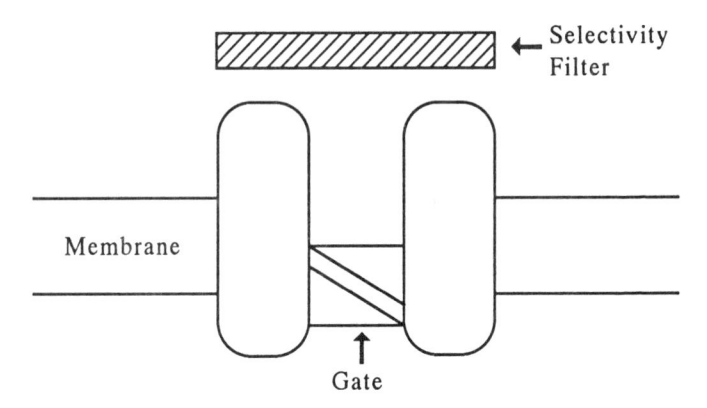

SODIUM. An *electrochemical gradient* draws sodium into the cell. Sodium, a positive ion, is attracted to the negative charge of the cell and would love to get away from the crowding of its cousins on the outside. This electrochemical gradient is a passive force and requires no energy to work. In fact, it can *provide* energy for the cell to use and does in a sodium-calcium exchange.

Active Forces

SODIUM-CALCIUM EXCHANGE. The wheeler-dealer cell uses energy derived from the sodium electrochemical gradient to expel calcium. The cell will take in three sodium ions to get rid of one calcium ion. This little trick is called the sodium-calcium exchange.

SODIUM-POTASSIUM PUMP. With the help of ATP and magnesium, the cell operates a sodium-potassium pump to push out sodium and suck potassium in. The pump helps restore the resting concentrations of sodium and potassium after the muscle contracts. (Digoxin blocks the action of this pump.)

CALCIUM-ATPase PUMP. The cell stores calcium in its reticulum. Sarcoplasmic reticulum (SR) is a network of fine tubules in the muscle cell.

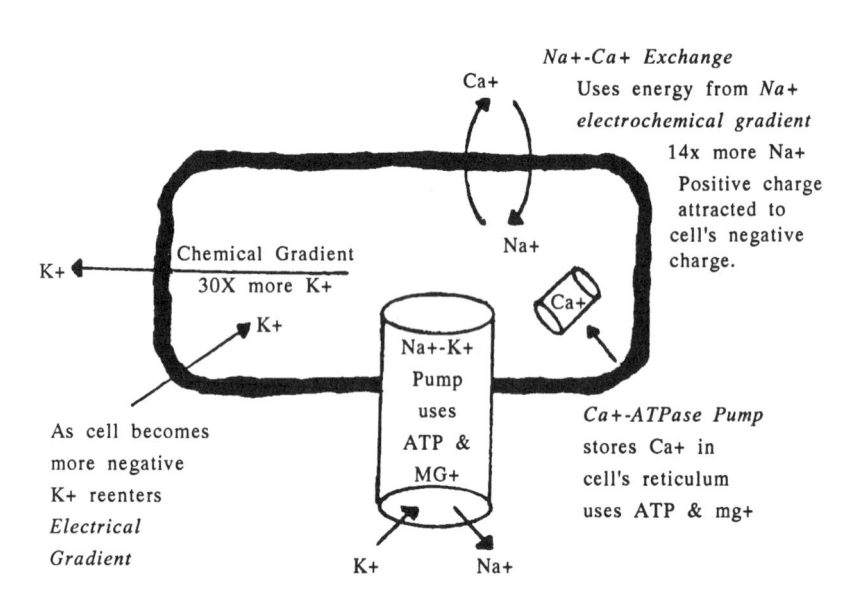

Na+-Ca+ Exchange
Uses energy from *Na+ electrochemical gradient*
14x more Na+
Positive charge attracted to cell's negative charge.

Ca+

Chemical Gradient
30X more K+

Na+

K+

K+

Ca+

Na+-K+ Pump uses ATP & MG+

As cell becomes more negative K+ reenters
Electrical Gradient

Ca+-ATPase Pump stores Ca+ in cell's reticulum uses ATP & mg+

K+   Na+

All this just to relax. Does it remind you of a day off from work?

DEPOLARIZATION AND CONTRACTION

Cells in the *sinus node,* the pacemaker of the heart, depolarize *automatically.* Their voltages do not remain negative in the resting phase but gradually become more positive over time. More research is needed to clarify why this happens. It is known that *slow calcium currents* are the major influence in the spontaneous depolarization of sinus node cells.

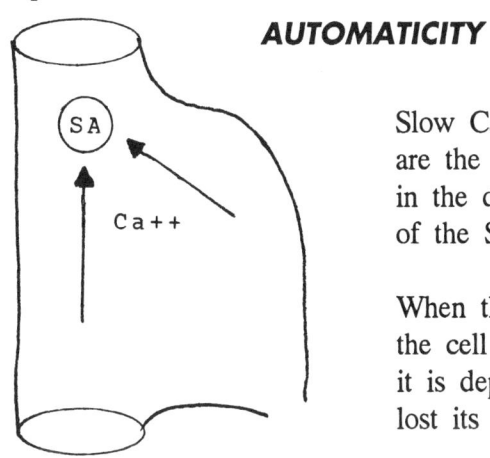

AUTOMATICITY

Slow Calcium Currents are the major influence in the depolarization of the SA node

When the interior of the cell becomes positive − it is depolarized - it has lost its negative edge

Once the sinus node depolarizes, the impulse spreads throughout the heart. The depolarization of one cell will spark its neighbors to follow suit.

To initiate depolarization *in the other cells,* a sodium channel will open its gate and *a fast sodium current* will rush the interior of the cell.

As the interior of the cell gains positive ions and the extracellular fluid loses them, the inside of the cell becomes positive for a *millisecond* and the extracellular fluid becomes negative.

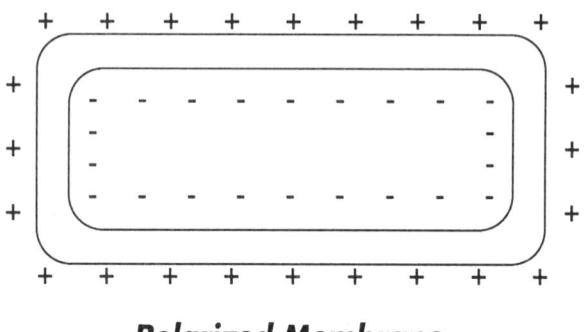

Polarized Membrane

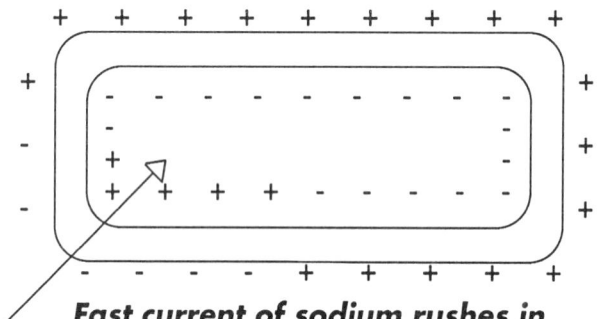

**Fast current of sodium rushes in
Depolarization Begins**

    The electrical signal generated by the rush of positive sodium ions triggers the release of *calcium* from the sarcoplasmic reticulum. Additionally, calcium channels in the cell wall open to allow in slow calcium currents.

    Calcium doesn't free-float inside the cell for long. It quickly binds with a protein called *troponin* found on the thin filament of the muscle. This bonding, in turn, stimulates another protein on the thin filament called *tropomyosin* to rotate in such a way that the muscle shortens. When a muscle shortens, it contracts.

Beta-adrenergic hormones, such as *epinephrine,* may increase inward calcium currents while *calcium channel blockers* hinder inward calcium movement. It is thought that when *digoxin* interferes with the sodium-potassium pump, the transmembrane sodium gradient decreases and less calcium is pumped out of the cell. The increased amounts of calcium available to the muscle increase its contractile strength.

The coupling of calcium to troponin alerts the cell to remove calcium and calcium removal mechanisms begin to work. As intracellular calcium levels decrease, the ion falls off troponin and the muscle lengthens and relaxes once again.

Immediately after depolarization, cardiac cells remain partly depolarized. This is called the *plateau period* and is unique to cardiac cells. It is a little insurance policy against tetanic contractions. During this time and in the initial stages of repolarization, the cell is *refractory* to further excitement.

In order to repolarize again, the cell must become negative again. Sodium ions, calcium ions and even potassium ions are sent away. Potassium, of course, will only be sent away in small numbers.

Just think how fast this happens. How often in a minute does your heart beat? Each time it has to depolarize, plateau, repolarize, depolarize ... We're talking fractions of a second here.

BIBLIOGRAPHY

Abedin Z. & Connnor R., *12 Lead ECG Interpretation: The Self Assessment Approach,* W. B. Saunders, Philadelphia, 1989.

Andreoli et al., *Comprehensive Cardiac Care,* C.V. Mosby, St. Louis, 6th Edition, 1987.

Chang, Raymond. *Chemistry,* Random House, New York, 2nd Edition, 1981

Chou, T.C., *Electrocardiography in Clinical Practice,* Mosby Year Book Inc. 2nd Edition, 1986.

Conover, M.B., *Understanding Electrocardiography,* C.V. Mosby, St. Louis 5th Edition, 1988.

Davis, Dale, *How to Quickly and Accurately Master ECG Interpretation,* Lippincott, Philadelphia, 1985.

Grauer K. and Curry C., *Clinical Electrocardiography,* Medical Economics Books, Blackwell Scientific Publications, Cambridge MA, 1987.

Flateland, Jill, *EKG Prep,* Center for Health Education, Arvada, Colorado

Marriott, J.L., *Practical Electrocardiography,* 8th Edition, Williams and Wilkins, Baltimore, 1988.

Marriott, H.J.L., *Pearls & Pitalls in Electrocardiography,* Lea & Febiger, Philadelphia 1990.

Marriott, J.L., *ECG: PDQ,* Williams and Wilkins, Baltimore 1987

Shoemaker et al., *Textbook of Critical Care,* Saunders, Philadelphia, 1989

Thome, Penelope, *Critical Care of the Acute MI,* Center for Health Education, Arvada, Colorado

Tortora G. and Anagnostakas N., *Principles of Anatomy and Physiology,* 4th Edition, Harper and Row, New York, 1984

Underhill et al., *Cardiac Nursing,* 2nd Edition, Lippincott, Philadelphia, 1989

Zipes and Jalife, *Cardiac Electrophysiology From Cell to Bedside,* W.B. Saunders, Philadelphia 1990

INDEX

Aberration
  Differential diagnosis — SVT with aberration from VT, 149
    alternating, 144
    atrial activity, 143
    AV dissociation, 150
    definition, 119, 142
    left bundle branch block, 120, 124, 125, 126
    morphology, 126
    preexisting bundle branch block and, 144
    right bundle branch block, 122, 123, 124
    triphasic contours, 143
Activation gate, 160
Adrenalin (epinephrine), 39, 165
Anterior infarction — See myocardial infarction
Arrowhead T waves, 76
Arteries
  AV nodal, 70, 72, 73, 120, 121
  circumflex, 69, 70-72, 85, 94
  diagonal, 70, 71
  left anterior descending, 69, 70-72, 85, 92, 93
  left main, 69-70
  posterior descending, 70-72, 96, 120
  ramis intermediary, 69, 70
  right coronary, 69, 70, 71, 86, 88, 95-97, 120
  septal perforators, 69, 70, 71, 120, 121
  sinus node artery, 70, 72, 73
Aortic insufficiency, 112
Aortic stenosis, 112

Atrial abnormality
  left, 111
  right, 110
Automaticity, 163
Axis
  defined, 56
  determination of, 55, 56
  deviation of
    anterior, 53
    causes, 58, 59
    left, 57, 137
    posterior, 53
    right, 55-57, 139
  indeterminate, 57
  no man's land, 57
  of a lead, 8

Bachman's Bundle, 24
Beta adrenergic hormones, 165
Bifasicular Block, 137
Bipolar leads
  definition, 8
  Einthoven's triangle, 20
  hexaxial reference, 20
Block
  bifasicular, 137
  bundle branch — See bundle branch block
  complicating myocardial infarction, 131
  fasicular, 136-140
Bundle, Bachman's, 24
Bundle Branches, 52, 58
  anatomy of, 26, 69, 120-121
  blood supply to, 69, 119-120
Bundle Branch Block, 119, 120, 126

INDEX

Bundle Branch Block *(continued)*
   causes of, 119, 124, 125
   critical rate and, 128
   diagnosis of myocardial infarction in
      the presence of, 131-134
      anterior wall, 132-134
      inferior wall, 133
   differential diagnosis from
      ventricular ectopy —
      See aberration
   intermittant, 119
   left, 124-127
   morphology, 126-127, 129, 130
   postdivisional, 125
   predivisional, 125
   rate dependent, 128
   right, 122-124, 127
   secondary ST-T changes with, 128-129
Bundle of HIS, 126

Calcium Channels, 164
Calcium Channel Blockers, 165
Cannon waves, 150
Cardiogenic shock, 92
Cerebral Bleeds, 37, 39
Chamber enlargement and hypertrophy
   — See hypertrophy
Changes
   indicative, 81, 82
   reciprocal, 81, 82
Channels
   calcium, 164
   phospholipid, 160
   protein, 160
Chemical gradient, 160

Chronic obstructive pulmonary disease,
   48, 52, 59, 109, 110, 139
Circumflex artery, 71, 85
Cornell voltage, 113-114
Complexes
   of aberration — see aberration
   biphasic, 41
   of bundle branch block —
      See bundle branch block
   concordance of, 148
   intervals and, 30-39
   labeling of, 30-39
   low voltage, 48
   negative — positive, 41, 43
   normal, 45-53
   P wave — see waves
   T wave — see waves
   QRS
      aberration, 147, 148
      bundle branch block and —
      See bundle branch block
      definition, 27
      labeling of, 34
      myocardial infarction and —
      See myocardial infarction
      ventricular ectopy and, 145-148
      transition, 52
   U wave — see waves
   ventricular, 145-148
   W waves — see waves
Concordance, 148
Conduction
   aberrant SVT vs VT —
      See aberration
   Bachman's bundle, 24
   bundle branches, 119

INDEX

Conduction *(continued)*
    channels — See channels
    definition, 24
    dipoles, 42
    electrolytes
        calcium, 24, 159, 161-165
        magnesium, 24, 161
        potassium, 24, 82, 158-162, 165
        sodium, 24, 158, 161-163, 165
    fasicles, 26
    nodes
        atrioventricular, 24-28, 33
        sinus, 24, 28, 163
Coronary artery
    left, 69
    right, 69, 71, 88
Coronary circulation, 69-73
Coving, 78
Critical rate, 128
Currents
    calcium, 163-164
    sodium, 163

Deflection, intrinsic, 42-43
Delta wave, 40
Depolarization, 24, 26, 157-165
    AV node, 24-27
    automaticity, 24, 163
    Bachman's bundle, 24
    bundle branches, 28
    calcium, 24, 159, 161-165
    channels, 164
    channel blockers, 165
    currents
        slow, 163
        fast, 163
    exchange, sodium-calcium, 161
    pump, calcium-ATPase, 162
    storage in cell, 161-162, 164-165
    chemical gradiant, 160
    currents
        calcium, 163
        fast, 163
        slow, 163
        sodium, 163
    digoxin, 161, 165
    electrochemical gradiant, 161
    exchange, sodium calcium, 161
    membrane potential, 159
    plateau period, 165
    potassium, 24, 82, 158-162, 165
    potential, 159
    Pump
        sodium-potassium, 161
        calcium-ATPase, 162
    Purkinje network, 27, 28
    SA node, 24, 28, 163
    sodium currents, 163
Deviation, axis — See axis
Dextrocardia, 58
Digoxin, 39, 161, 165
Dipole, 42
Dissociation, AV, 150
Drugs
    Digoxin, 39, 161, 165
    calcium channel blockers, 165
    epinephrine, 39, 165
    quinidine, 39

Early repolarization, 99
Ectopy
    morphology, ventricular, 145-148

INDEX

Ectopy *(continued)*
    ventricular versus SVT with aberration — See aberration
Einthoven's triangle, 20
Electrocardiogram
    graph paper, 31-32
    normal left-sided, 45-53, 60
    normal right-sided, 90
Electrochemical gradients, 161
Embolism, 55
Emphysema (COPD), 48, 52, 59, 109, 110, 139
Enlargement — See hypertrophy
Epinephrine, 39, 165
Exchange, sodium-calcium, 161, 162
Exercise, 39

Failure, cardiac, 48
Fasicles, 26, 69, 120-121
Fasicular block — See hemiblock
Fast sodium currents, 163
Fibrous skeleton, 119
Fireman's hat, 77
Frontal plane leads, 9-14, 20-22, 45-47

Graph, EKG, 31-32

Hemiblock, 136, 137, 138
    alternate terms for, 136, 138
    bifasicular, 137
    diagnostic criteria for, 137, 140
        anterior, 136-137, 140
        posterior, 138-140
Hexaxial reference system, 20, 21, 55
HIS bundle, 26

Horizontal plane leads, 22
Hypertension
    pulmonic, 112, 116
    systemic, 33, 92
Hypertrophy, 108, 109
    atrial, left, 111
    atrial, right, 110
    strain, 114, 117
    ventricular, left, 27, 58, 112
    ventricular, right, 58, 112, 115-117
Hypotension, 89, 95

Imbalances, electrolyte, 37, 38
Indeterminate axis, 57
Infarction — See myocardial infarction
Inferior wall MI — See myocardial infarction
Injury, pattern of, 75-79
Ischemia, 75, 76
Intrinsic deflection, 43

J joint, 33, 36
Jugular venous distention, 89

Kussmal's sign, 89

Leads
    I, 9, 20-22, 45
    II, 9, 10, 20-22, 45
    III, 9, 11, 20-22, 46
    aVF, 9, 14, 22, 46
    aVL, 9, 13, 22, 46
    aVR, 9, 12, 22, 46
    bipolar, 8
    in hexaxial reference, 20, 21

INDEX

Leads *(continued)*
    limb, 11, 12, 45
    MCL_1, 19, 142
    orphan, 12
    precordial, 14, 16
    right ventricular, 17, 18
    unipolar, 8, 9, 11, 12, 14
    V leads, 9, 14, 22, 48-50
Left anterior hemiblock (LAHB) —
    See hemiblock
Left axis deviation, 57
Left bundle branch —
    See Bundle Branch
Left bundle branch block —
    See bundle branch block
Left coronary artery, 69-70
Left posterior hemiblock —
    See hemiblock
Left ventricular hypertrophy —
    See hypertrophy
Left ventricular pattern, 53
Low voltage, 48

MCL_1, 19, 142
MCL_6, 142
Mean cardiac vector, 29, 55
Membrane potential, 159
Mirror test, 88, 96
Mobitz type II 2° AV block, 85, 92
Morphology of ventricular complexes
    — See aberration
Myocardial infarction, 37
    anterior wall, 71, 85, 92, 134
    atrial, 91
    complicated by bundle branch
      block, 131-134

    complications, 92-97
    evolution of, 82-83
    indicative changes in, 81
    ischemia, pattern of, 75, 76
    inferior, 58, 71, 85, 86, 95, 133
    injury, pattern of, 75-79
    lateral wall, 58, 71, 85, 94, 139
    necrosis, pattern, 75
    posterior, 71, 86, 96
    Q wave in, 75-76, 79-83
    Q wave versus non-Q wave, 80
    reciprocal changes in, 81
    right ventricular, 88-90, 97
    septal, 93
    stages of, 82
    ST segment, 75-102
    T wave, 75, 76, 77, 75-102

Necrosis, patterns of, 75
Net vector, 29
Neutral reference point, 11
Nodes — See conduction, Nodes
No man's land, 57
Non-Q wave infarction, 80
Normal EKG, 45-53, 90
Notching, 40

Obesity, 48, 52, 109
Orphan lead, 12

P mitral, 32, 111
P pulmonale, 32, 110
P wave, 25, 27, 32, 33, 45-53
Patterns
    of injury, 75
    of ischemia, 75-76

INDEX

Patterns *(continued)*
  left ventricular, 50
  of necrosis, 75
  right ventricular, 48
Pericardial effusion, 48
Pericarditis
  EKG changes, 98, 102
  signs and symptoms, 98
  stages, 100-103
PR interval (PRI), 27, 33, 40
Plateau period, 165
Posterior wall MI —
  See myocardial infarction
Potassium, 24, 82, 158-162, 165
Potential, 159
Pregnancy, 58
Pulmonary embolus, 55, 58
Purkinje network, 27, 28
Pump
  calcium-ATPase, 162
  sodium-potassium, 161

Q wave — See QRS complex, Q wave
QT interval, 37, 38
QRS complex, 27, 34, 36, 39, 42
  axis determination, 55-57
  delta wave and, 40
  in left bundle branch block —
    See bundle branch block
  in ventricular hypertrophy —
    See hypertrophy
  in normal EKG, 45-53
  in right bundle branch block —
    See bundle branch block
  left ventricular pattern
  notching of, 40

Q wave in
  description of, 34-35
  in left bundle branch block, 133
  in horizontal hearts, 47
  in myocardial infarction, 75-76, 79-83
  in vertical hearts, 47
  normal, 45-53
  septal, 53
Right ventricular pattern, 51
R wave in
  description of, 34-35
  in hemiblock (fasicular block), 140
  in left bundle branch block, 129
  in normal EKG, 45-53
  in right bundle branch bock, 123, 129
  progression of in V leads, 52
S wave in
  description of, 34-35
  in hemiblock (fasicular block), 140
  in left bundle branch block, 129
  in normal EKG, 45-53
  in right bundle branch block, 123, 129
  slurring of, 39
QS complex, 35, 85, 93
Quinidine, 39

RAA: Right atrial abnormality —
  See hypertrophy
RBB: Right bundle branch block —
  See bundle branch block

INDEX

RVH: Right ventricular hypertrophy — See hypertrophy
R wave — See QRS complex, R wave
Rabbit ears
   in right bundle branch block, 123
   in ventricular ectopy, 145
Ramus intermedius artery — See arteries
Repolarization, early, 99
Resting membrane potential, 159
Reticulum, sarcoplasmic, 159
Right axis deviation, 57
R wave progression, 52

S wave — See QRS complex, S wave
SA node, 24, 28
Segment
   PR, 34, 91
   QT, 37-38
   ST
      definition, 36
      depression of, 76, 77
      elevation, 75, 77
      frowning, 78
      secondary to BBB, 129
      shape of, 36
      smiling, 78, 100, 102
   TP, 100
Selectivity filters, 160
Sensitivity, 113
Shock, 89
Sinoatrial (SA) node, 24, 28, 163
Sinus node artery, 70, 72, 73
Sinuses of Valsalva, 69
Slow calcium currents, 163

Sodium, 24, 158, 161-163, 165
Specificity, 113
ST segment — See segment, ST
Strain pattern
   in left ventricular hypertrophy, 114
   in right ventricular hypertrophy, 115, 117
Stenosis
   aortic, 112
   pulmonic, 110, 116
Subendocardial infarction, 80
Sudden death, 37
Summation gallop, 89
Syncope, 37

T wave, 27, 29, 37
   causes of changes, 76
   coving, 78
   fireman's hat, 77
   hyperacute, 82
   inversion, 76
   ischemia, 76
   in left ventricular hypertrophy, 114
   normal, 39, 45-53
   primary, 128
   secondary to bundle branch block, 128, 129, 130
   ST segment and — See Segment, ST
   strain and, 114, 115, 117
   tombstone T, 77
Tetralogy of Fallot, 112, 116
Third Degree AV block, 92
Time and voltage measurements, 31-32
Torsades de Points, 37
Transposition of great vessels, 112

INDEX

Tropomysin, 164
Troponin, 164
Transition zone, 52
Tricuspid insufficiency, 112

U wave, 27, 29
Unipolar leads — See leads, unipolar

Valsalva, sinuses of, 69
Vector(s)
  definition, 25
  mean cardiac, 29
Ventricular ectopy
  morphology, 145, 146-148
  myths, 149
  versus aberration — See aberration
Ventricular gallop, 89
Ventricular hypertrophy —
  See hypertrophy
Ventricular reentry tachycardia, 37
Voltage
  low, 48
  negative, 41
  positive, 41

W wave
Walls
  anterior
    leads, 15, 16
    in myocardial infarction —
      See myocardial infarction
  inferior
    leads, 10, 11, 14
    in myocardial infarction —
      See myocardial infarction
  lateral
    leads, 9, 13, 16
    in myocardial infarction —
      See myocardial infarction
  posterior
    leads, 86-87
    in myocardial infarction —
      See myocardial infarction
  right ventricular
    leads, 18, 88
    in myocardial infarction —
      See myocardial infarction
Waves
  delta, 40
  P wave, 27, 32
    abnormal, 32, 110
    definition, 25
    increased amplitude, 32, 110
    increased width, 110
    notching, 32, 110
    peaking, 110
  Q wave — See QRS complex,
    Q wave
  R wave — See QRS complex,
    R wave
  T wave — See T wave
  U wave, 27, 29, 37, 39
  W waves, 133
Wolf-parkinson White, 40, 59

Zone, transition, 52

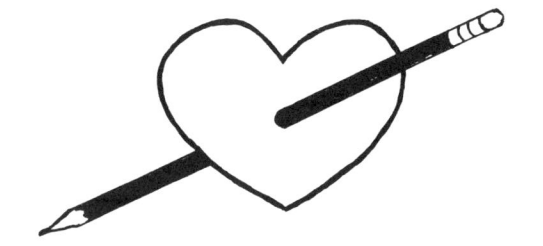

CEU EXAM

CEU EXAM

TAKE THIS TEST - and earn CEU's! Do not write on the test questions as this CEU exam may be shared with your friends.

INSTRUCTIONS:

At the end of this book are answer sheets with an evaluation form. Write your answer in the corresponding box on the answer form.

Be sure to complete the evaluation form located on the back of the answer sheets.

Cut out answer sheet/evaluation form only (keep the test) and mail it to: CEU Access, 20 Camelot Road, Parsippany, NJ 07054. A $10.00 processing fee is required for each test. Send a check or money order payable to CEU Access. In 4 weeks you will be notified of your test results. Upon passing the test a certificate for 6.5 contact hours (0.65 CEU's from the American Association of Critical Care Nurses in category A) will be awarded. If you fail the test you have the option of taking the test again at no cost.

DO NOT WRITE ON TEST QUESTIONS, USE ANSWER SHEET

CEU EXAM
LEADS

1. The bipolar leads are:
   a. aVR, aVL, aVF
   b. V_1, V_2, V_3
   c. I, II, III

2. Some unipolar leads are:
   a. I, II, III
   b. aVR, aVL, aVF
   c. I, II, V_3

3. Lead I records the electrical activity between:
   a. the right arm and the left arm
   b. the right arm and the left foot
   c. the left foot and the right arm

4. The direct path between two electrodes or between one electrode and a neutral reference point is called:
   a. a lead
   b. an axis

5. Lead II looks at:
   a. the lateral wall
   b. the inferior wall
   c. the anterior wall

6. Which lead has the positive electrode on the left leg and the negative electrode on the right shoulder?
   a. I
   b. II
   c. III

7. The inferior wall of the heart can be viewed in which limb-lead inferior wall watchers?
   a. II, III, aVL
   b. I, aVL
   c. II, III, aVF

177

DO NOT WRITE ON TEST QUESTIONS, USE ANSWER SHEET

8. Which are the unipolar limb leads?
   a. I, II, III, aVR, aVL, aVF
   b. V_1, V_6, aVR, aVL, aVF
   c. V_1, V_2, V_3, V_4, V_5, V_6
   d. aVR, aVL, aVF

9. Which leads look at the lateral wall of the heart?
   a. I, aVL
   b. I, aVF
   c. II, aVL

10. The chest leads view the heart
    a. in a frontal plane
    b. in a horizontal plane
    c. in a DC-10 plane

11. Which of the anterior leads examine the septum?
    a. V_3, V_4
    b. $V_1 - V_4$
    c. V_1, V_2

12. Leads V_1 through V_6 look at the:
    a. anterior and inferior wall
    b. anterior and lateral wall
    c. septum and anterior wall
    d. septum, anterior and lateral wall

13. MCL_1, mimics:
    a. V_1
    b. V_6

14. MCL_1, a good lead for constant monitoring, has its positive electrode:
    a. on the right shoulder
    b. on the left shoulder
    c. at the 4th intercostal space, right of the sternum
    d. at the 4th intercostal space, left of the sternum

DO NOT WRITE ON TEST QUESTIONS, USE ANSWER SHEET

15. Hexaxial reference is a system in which:
    a. all frontal leads lie in precise relation to each other
    b. all horizontal leads lie in precise relation to each other

CONDUCTION

16. Conduction time through the AV node
    a. slows to a crawl
    b. speeds up

17. The left bundle branch depolarizes _____ the right bundle branch
    a. after
    b. before

18. Conduction time through the Purkinje fibers:
    a. is fast
    b. is slow

19. The PRI represents the electrical impulse travelling through the AV node, the bundle of HIS, the bundle branches and the Purkinje fibers
    a. true
    b. false

20. The QRS represents ventricular systole
    a. true
    b. false

21. The U wave represents atrial relaxation
    a. true
    b. false

DO NOT WRITE ON TEST QUESTIONS, USE ANSWER SHEET

COMPLEXES AND INTERVALS

22. A normal P wave had a rounded shape and it does not exceed
    a. 0.05 secs
    b. 0.20 secs
    c. 0.11 secs

23. A normal PR interval is
    a. 0.05 to 0.11 secs
    b. 0.12 to 0.20 secs
    c. 0.05 to 0.20 secs

24. The first negative deflection in a QRS complex is
    a. P wave
    b. S wave
    c. Q wave
    d. QRS complex

25. The negative deflection that follows the R wave is
    a. a Q wave
    b. an R wave
    c. an S wave

26. The QRS complex normally ranges from
    a. 0.05 to 0.11 secs
    b. 0.05 to 0.20 secs
    c. 0.05 to 0.13 secs

27. The ST segment represents the time between ventricular contraction and relaxation
    a. true
    b. false

DO NOT WRITE ON TEST QUESTIONS, USE ANSWER SHEET

28. The QT interval measures the time it takes for the ventricles to contract and relax
    a. true
    b. false

29. The ST segment is normally above or below the isoelectric line
    a. true
    b. false

30. Prolonged QT intervals are associated with ventricular reentry tachycardia
    a. true
    b. false

31. Delayed relaxation of the ventricles is represented by short QT intervals
    a. true
    b. false

32. The U wave is generally of the same polarity as the preceeding T wave
    a. true
    b. false

33. When an electrical current travels toward an electrode, it draws a negative complex
    a. true
    b. false

DO NOT WRITE ON TEST QUESTIONS, USE ANSWER SHEET

34. When an electrical current travels away from an electrode, it draws a negative complex
    a. true
    b. false

NORMAL EKG

35. Which complexes are normally upright?
    a. I, II, aVR
    b. II, III, aVR
    c. I, II, aVF

36. The lead that normally shows negative complexes is
    a. aVL
    b. aVR
    c. aVF

37. If the heart has a vertical axis, small Q waves are likely to be found in
    a. II, III, and aVF
    b. I and aVL

38. If the heart has a more horizontal axis, small Q waves are likely to be found in
    a. II, III, and aVF
    b. I and aVL

39. A QRS wearing lingerie is
    a. normal
    b. probably not normal but probably not slurred, either

DO NOT WRITE ON TEST QUESTIONS, USE ANSWER SHEET

40. T waves in the limb leads should not exceed
    a. 3 mm
    b. 5 mm
    c. 10 mm
    d. 12 mm

41. A small R wave is V_6 is
    a. normal
    b. abnormal

42. The normal transition phase is
    a. between V_1 and V_2
    b. between V_3 and V_4
    c. between V_5 and V_6

43. T waves in the chest leads should not exceed
    a. 3 mm
    b. 5 mm
    c. 10 mm
    d. 12 mm

ARTERIAL PERFUSION

44. The left ventricular free wall receives its blood supply from the
    a. circumflex
    b. LAD
    c. left main coronary artery

DO NOT WRITE ON TEST QUESTIONS, USE ANSWER SHEET

45. Branches of the LAD called septal perforating arteries perfuse the
    a. posterior 1/3 of the interventricular septum
    b. anterior 1/3 of the interventricular septum
    c. anterior 2/3 of the interventricular septum

46. The main trunk of the right bundle branch and both major fasicles of the left bundle branch nestle in the
    a. posterior 1/3 of the interventricular septum
    b. anterior 1/3 of the interventricular septum
    c. anterior 2/3 of the interventricular septum

47. The left circumflex artery gives its blood to the
    a. anterior wall
    b. lateral wall
    c. inferior wall

48. In 90% of hearts, the right coronary artery gives rise to the
    a. posterior descending artery
    b. ramus intermedius

49. The posterior descending artery has septal perforating branches that perfuse the
    a. posterior 1/3 of the interventricular septum
    b. anterior 1/3 of the interventricular septum
    c. anterior 2/3 of the interventricular septum

50. Occlusion of the RCA results in
    a. inferior wall infarction
    b. posterior wall infarction
    c. lateral wall infarction
    d. a and b
    e. b and c

DO NOT WRITE ON TEST QUESTIONS, USE ANSWER SHEET

51. In 90% of hearts a branch of the RCA forms
    a. the SA nodal artery
    b. the AV nodal artery
    c. a and b

52. An occlusion of the LAD could result in
    a. inferior wall damage
    b. septal wall damage
    c. anterior and lateral wall damage
    d. b and c

53. If your patient has major disease in all the main arteries, what keeps the patient alive?
    a. the nurse
    b. collateral circulation
    c. the doctor
    d. a and b
    e. all of the above

LANDSCAPE OF MI

54. An EKG shows ischemia as
    a. a Q wave
    b. ST elevation
    c. inverted T waves

55. ST elevation
    a. is always abnormal
    b. in a coved shape usually means injury
    c. is always normal

56. Q waves that are greater than one baby box wide or are 25% of the R wave deep
    a. signify necrotic tissue
    b. are normal in certain leads

DO NOT WRITE ON TEST QUESTIONS, USE ANSWER SHEET

INFARCTION, WALL TO WALL

57. If a patient's EKG shows ST elevation in leads V_1, V2, and V3, this would indicate
    a. anterior wall ischemia
    b. lateral wall ischemia
    c. anterior wall injury

58. When reviewing your patient's 12-lead EKG, you notice deep and wide Q waves in 1, aVL, V_4, V_5 and V_6, you suspect
    a. anterior wall MI
    b. lateral wall MI
    c. inferior wall MI

59. Reciprocal changes for the inferior wall are seen in
    a. leads II, III, and aVF
    b. leads I and aVL
    c. V_1, V_2, and V_3

60. Which wall can you use the mirror test on?
    a. posterior wall
    b. anterior wall
    c. lateral wall

61. Suspect a posterior wall infarct when
    a. when tall R waves are present in V_1 and/or V_2
    b. there are no R waves present in the entire EKG
    c. when it doesn't fit in any other category

DO NOT WRITE ON TEST QUESTIONS, USE ANSWER SHEET

PERICARDITIS

62. The initial stage of pericarditis shows
    a. ST elevations in many leads
    b. ST elevations in leads II, III, and aVF only

63. New Q waves will appear on the EKG with pericarditis
    a. true
    b. false

VENTRICULAR HYPERTROPHY AND BUNDLE BRANCH BLOCK

64. Tall peaked P waves in the inferior leads mean
    a. left atrial abnormalities
    b. right atrial abnormalities

65. Wide Dolly Parton P waves greater than 0.04 seconds could suggest
    a. atrial hypertrophy from mitral stenosis or mitral insuffiency
    b. your patient is from the south

66. Leads that show strain in the left ventricle are:
    a. I, AVL, V_5, V_6
    b. V_1, V_2

DO NOT WRITE ON TEST QUESTIONS, USE ANSWER SHEET

67. Activities of the left ventricle usually control the EKG stylus
    a. true
    b. false

68. Symmetrical T wave inversion in leads I, aVL, V_5, V_6 mean left ventricular strain
    a. true
    b. false

69. Right ventricular strain show the same ST depressions and T wave inversions in leads
    a. II, III, aVF, V_1, V_2
    b. I, aVL, V_5, V_6

BUNDLE BRANCH BLOCK

70. Both right and left BBB will show changes in leads V_1 and V_6
    a. true
    b. false
71. The "rabbit" ear complex is characteristic of the RBBB
    a. true
    b. false
72. The wide slurred S wave is seen in RBBB in lead V_6
    a. true
    b. false

DO NOT WRITE ON TEST QUESTIONS, USE ANSWER SHEET

73. Normal depolarization takes place in LBBB
    a. true
    b. false

74. LBBB has a characteristic R wave which is notched and slurred in leads I and V_6
    a. true
    b. false

75. A LBBB has a positive QRS complex in V_1 and V_6
    a. true
    b. false

76. The QRS complex is greater than 0.11 in a BBB
    a. true
    b. false

77. Secondary T wave changes in a BBB are
    a. normal
    b. abnormal

BBB & MI

78. The diagnosis of an MI in the face of a LBBB is a pain in the neck:
    a. true
    b. false

79. Q waves with a LBBB of 0.04 seconds or longer in leads I, V_5 and V_6
    a. quietly discuss MI
    b. shout out MI
    c. are normal

DO NOT WRITE ON TEST QUESTIONS, USE ANSWER SHEET

HEMIBLOCKS

80. A hemiblock refers to either the blockage of:
    a. the right bundle branch or the left bundle branch
    b. the left anterior fasicle or the left posterior fasicle

81. The left anterior fasicle is supplied by:
    a. the LAD
    b. the RCA
    c. the LAD and the RCA

82. Left posterior hemiblock results in:
    a. right axis deviation
    b. left axis deviation

83. Left posterior hemiblock is common if right bundle branch block is also present
    a. true
    b. false

ABERRATION AND ECTOPY

84. Aberration is like a temporary
    a. BBB
    b. SVT
    c. VT

85. The best lead for constant observation is:
    a. II
    b. MCL_1
    c. MCL_6

DO NOT WRITE ON TEST QUESTIONS, USE ANSWER SHEET

86. You can change an MCL_1 into an MCL_6 by moving the positive electrode to the
    a. 4th intercoastal space at the right sternal border
    b. to the 4th intercoastal space at the midclavicular line
    c. to the 5th intercoastal space at the left anterior axillary line

87. Aberration is more common than ectopy
    a. true
    b. false

88. Triphasic contours of rsR´ in V_1 speak in favor of aberration
    a. true
    b. false

89. The complex of right ventricular ectopy is negative in V1
    a. true
    b. false

90. The complex of left ventricular ectopy is positive in V_1
    a. true
    b. false

91. Ventricular ectopy assumes favorite silhouettes in certain leads — it is best to memorize them
    a. true
    b. false

DO NOT WRITE ON TEST QUESTIONS, USE ANSWER SHEET

92. If the rabbit's _____ ear is taller, it speaks in favor of ectopy:
    a. left
    b. right

93. A monphasic QS with a slurred upstroke in V_1 speaks for:
    a. ectopy
    b. aberration

94. A monophasic QS with a slurred downstroke in V_1 speaks for:
    a. ectopy
    b. aberration

95. Both SVT and VT can be regular rhythms:
    a. true
    b. false

96. Both SVT and VT can be well tolerated for hours:
    a. true
    b. false

97. A good question to ask a patient sitting in bed, reading the paper under a monitor with a lethal rhythm is:
    a. What's good in the paper?
    b. When did you notice your heart beating fast?

ANSWER FORM
See instructions on page 176

1.	a ☐	b ☐	c ☐	d ☐	e ☐	50.	a ☐	b ☐	c ☐	d ☐	e ☐
2.	a ☐	b ☐	c ☐	d ☐	e ☐	51.	a ☐	b ☐	c ☐	d ☐	e ☐
3.	a ☐	b ☐	c ☐	d ☐	e ☐	52.	a ☐	b ☐	c ☐	d ☐	e ☐
4.	a ☐	b ☐	c ☐	d ☐	e ☐	53.	a ☐	b ☐	c ☐	d ☐	e ☐
5.	a ☐	b ☐	c ☐	d ☐	e ☐	54.	a ☐	b ☐	c ☐	d ☐	e ☐
6.	a ☐	b ☐	c ☐	d ☐	e ☐	55.	a ☐	b ☐	c ☐	d ☐	e ☐
7.	a ☐	b ☐	c ☐	d ☐	e ☐	56.	a ☐	b ☐	c ☐	d ☐	e ☐
8.	a ☐	b ☐	c ☐	d ☐	e ☐	57.	a ☐	b ☐	c ☐	d ☐	e ☐
9.	a ☐	b ☐	c ☐	d ☐	e ☐	58.	a ☐	b ☐	c ☐	d ☐	e ☐
10.	a ☐	b ☐	c ☐	d ☐	e ☐	59.	a ☐	b ☐	c ☐	d ☐	e ☐
11.	a ☐	b ☐	c ☐	d ☐	e ☐	60.	a ☐	b ☐	c ☐	d ☐	e ☐
12.	a ☐	b ☐	c ☐	d ☐	e ☐	61.	a ☐	b ☐	c ☐	d ☐	e ☐
13.	a ☐	b ☐	c ☐	d ☐	e ☐	62.	a ☐	b ☐	c ☐	d ☐	e ☐
14.	a ☐	b ☐	c ☐	d ☐	e ☐	63.	a ☐	b ☐	c ☐	d ☐	e ☐
15.	a ☐	b ☐	c ☐	d ☐	e ☐	64.	a ☐	b ☐	c ☐	d ☐	e ☐
16.	a ☐	b ☐	c ☐	d ☐	e ☐	65.	a ☐	b ☐	c ☐	d ☐	e ☐
17.	a ☐	b ☐	c ☐	d ☐	e ☐	66.	a ☐	b ☐	c ☐	d ☐	e ☐
18.	a ☐	b ☐	c ☐	d ☐	e ☐	67.	a ☐	b ☐	c ☐	d ☐	e ☐
19.	a ☐	b ☐	c ☐	d ☐	e ☐	68.	a ☐	b ☐	c ☐	d ☐	e ☐
20.	a ☐	b ☐	c ☐	d ☐	e ☐	69.	a ☐	b ☐	c ☐	d ☐	e ☐
21.	a ☐	b ☐	c ☐	d ☐	e ☐	70.	a ☐	b ☐	c ☐	d ☐	e ☐
22.	a ☐	b ☐	c ☐	d ☐	e ☐	71.	a ☐	b ☐	c ☐	d ☐	e ☐
23.	a ☐	b ☐	c ☐	d ☐	e ☐	72.	a ☐	b ☐	c ☐	d ☐	e ☐
24.	a ☐	b ☐	c ☐	d ☐	e ☐	73.	a ☐	b ☐	c ☐	d ☐	e ☐
25.	a ☐	b ☐	c ☐	d ☐	e ☐	74.	a ☐	b ☐	c ☐	d ☐	e ☐
26.	a ☐	b ☐	c ☐	d ☐	e ☐	75.	a ☐	b ☐	c ☐	d ☐	e ☐
27.	a ☐	b ☐	c ☐	d ☐	e ☐	76.	a ☐	b ☐	c ☐	d ☐	e ☐
28.	a ☐	b ☐	c ☐	d ☐	e ☐	77.	a ☐	b ☐	c ☐	d ☐	e ☐
29.	a ☐	b ☐	c ☐	d ☐	e ☐	78.	a ☐	b ☐	c ☐	d ☐	e ☐
30.	a ☐	b ☐	c ☐	d ☐	e ☐	79.	a ☐	b ☐	c ☐	d ☐	e ☐
31.	a ☐	b ☐	c ☐	d ☐	e ☐	80.	a ☐	b ☐	c ☐	d ☐	e ☐
32.	a ☐	b ☐	c ☐	d ☐	e ☐	81.	a ☐	b ☐	c ☐	d ☐	e ☐
33.	a ☐	b ☐	c ☐	d ☐	e ☐	82.	a ☐	b ☐	c ☐	d ☐	e ☐
34.	a ☐	b ☐	c ☐	d ☐	e ☐	83.	a ☐	b ☐	c ☐	d ☐	e ☐
35.	a ☐	b ☐	c ☐	d ☐	e ☐	84.	a ☐	b ☐	c ☐	d ☐	e ☐
36.	a ☐	b ☐	c ☐	d ☐	e ☐	85.	a ☐	b ☐	c ☐	d ☐	e ☐
37.	a ☐	b ☐	c ☐	d ☐	e ☐	86.	a ☐	b ☐	c ☐	d ☐	e ☐
38.	a ☐	b ☐	c ☐	d ☐	e ☐	87.	a ☐	b ☐	c ☐	d ☐	e ☐
39.	a ☐	b ☐	c ☐	d ☐	e ☐	88.	a ☐	b ☐	c ☐	d ☐	e ☐
40.	a ☐	b ☐	c ☐	d ☐	e ☐	89.	a ☐	b ☐	c ☐	d ☐	e ☐
41.	a ☐	b ☐	c ☐	d ☐	e ☐	90.	a ☐	b ☐	c ☐	d ☐	e ☐
42.	a ☐	b ☐	c ☐	d ☐	e ☐	91.	a ☐	b ☐	c ☐	d ☐	e ☐
43.	a ☐	b ☐	c ☐	d ☐	e ☐	92.	a ☐	b ☐	c ☐	d ☐	e ☐
44.	a ☐	b ☐	c ☐	d ☐	e ☐	93.	a ☐	b ☐	c ☐	d ☐	e ☐
45.	a ☐	b ☐	c ☐	d ☐	e ☐	94.	a ☐	b ☐	c ☐	d ☐	e ☐
46.	a ☐	b ☐	c ☐	d ☐	e ☐	95.	a ☐	b ☐	c ☐	d ☐	e ☐
47.	a ☐	b ☐	c ☐	d ☐	e ☐	96.	a ☐	b ☐	c ☐	d ☐	e ☐
48.	a ☐	b ☐	c ☐	d ☐	e ☐	97.	a ☐	b ☐	c ☐	d ☐	e ☐
49.	a ☐	b ☐	c ☐	d ☐	e ☐						

EVALUATION OF TEXT AND TEST

Name: _____

Address: _____

City: _____ State: _____

Phone: (____) _____ ZIP: _____

Occupation: RN ☐   LPN ☐   EMT ☐
             Paramedic ☐   Other _____

License # _____ State _____

Soc.Sec.# _____

How many hours did it take you to read the book and take the test: _____ hrs.

Did you find the material presented: *check all that apply*

☐ excellent   ☐ clear   ☐ well organized

☐ good   ☐ interesting   ☐ poorly organized

☐ fair   ☐ dull   ☐ too long

☐ poor   ☐ confusing   ☐ too short

Was the CEU test? *check all that apply*

☐ too hard   ☐ too long

☐ too easy   ☐ too short   ☐ about right

Thank you for your time. Any comments you would like to make are welcome. Any recommendation/suggestions for the 2nd edition would be appreciated.

ANSWER FORM
See instructions on page 176

	a	b	c	d	e			a	b	c	d	e
1.	☐	☐	☐	☐	☐		50.	☐	☐	☐	☐	☐
2.	☐	☐	☐	☐	☐		51.	☐	☐	☐	☐	☐
3.	☐	☐	☐	☐	☐		52.	☐	☐	☐	☐	☐
4.	☐	☐	☐	☐	☐		53.	☐	☐	☐	☐	☐
5.	☐	☐	☐	☐	☐		54.	☐	☐	☐	☐	☐
6.	☐	☐	☐	☐	☐		55.	☐	☐	☐	☐	☐
7.	☐	☐	☐	☐	☐		56.	☐	☐	☐	☐	☐
8.	☐	☐	☐	☐	☐		57.	☐	☐	☐	☐	☐
9.	☐	☐	☐	☐	☐		58.	☐	☐	☐	☐	☐
10.	☐	☐	☐	☐	☐		59.	☐	☐	☐	☐	☐
11.	☐	☐	☐	☐	☐		60.	☐	☐	☐	☐	☐
12.	☐	☐	☐	☐	☐		61.	☐	☐	☐	☐	☐
13.	☐	☐	☐	☐	☐		62.	☐	☐	☐	☐	☐
14.	☐	☐	☐	☐	☐		63.	☐	☐	☐	☐	☐
15.	☐	☐	☐	☐	☐		64.	☐	☐	☐	☐	☐
16.	☐	☐	☐	☐	☐		65.	☐	☐	☐	☐	☐
17.	☐	☐	☐	☐	☐		66.	☐	☐	☐	☐	☐
18.	☐	☐	☐	☐	☐		67.	☐	☐	☐	☐	☐
19.	☐	☐	☐	☐	☐		68.	☐	☐	☐	☐	☐
20.	☐	☐	☐	☐	☐		69.	☐	☐	☐	☐	☐
21.	☐	☐	☐	☐	☐		70.	☐	☐	☐	☐	☐
22.	☐	☐	☐	☐	☐		71.	☐	☐	☐	☐	☐
23.	☐	☐	☐	☐	☐		72.	☐	☐	☐	☐	☐
24.	☐	☐	☐	☐	☐		73.	☐	☐	☐	☐	☐
25.	☐	☐	☐	☐	☐		74.	☐	☐	☐	☐	☐
26.	☐	☐	☐	☐	☐		75.	☐	☐	☐	☐	☐
27.	☐	☐	☐	☐	☐		76.	☐	☐	☐	☐	☐
28.	☐	☐	☐	☐	☐		77.	☐	☐	☐	☐	☐
29.	☐	☐	☐	☐	☐		78.	☐	☐	☐	☐	☐
30.	☐	☐	☐	☐	☐		79.	☐	☐	☐	☐	☐
31.	☐	☐	☐	☐	☐		80.	☐	☐	☐	☐	☐
32.	☐	☐	☐	☐	☐		81.	☐	☐	☐	☐	☐
33.	☐	☐	☐	☐	☐		82.	☐	☐	☐	☐	☐
34.	☐	☐	☐	☐	☐		83.	☐	☐	☐	☐	☐
35.	☐	☐	☐	☐	☐		84.	☐	☐	☐	☐	☐
36.	☐	☐	☐	☐	☐		85.	☐	☐	☐	☐	☐
37.	☐	☐	☐	☐	☐		86.	☐	☐	☐	☐	☐
38.	☐	☐	☐	☐	☐		87.	☐	☐	☐	☐	☐
39.	☐	☐	☐	☐	☐		88.	☐	☐	☐	☐	☐
40.	☐	☐	☐	☐	☐		89.	☐	☐	☐	☐	☐
41.	☐	☐	☐	☐	☐		90.	☐	☐	☐	☐	☐
42.	☐	☐	☐	☐	☐		91.	☐	☐	☐	☐	☐
43.	☐	☐	☐	☐	☐		92.	☐	☐	☐	☐	☐
44.	☐	☐	☐	☐	☐		93.	☐	☐	☐	☐	☐
45.	☐	☐	☐	☐	☐		94.	☐	☐	☐	☐	☐
46.	☐	☐	☐	☐	☐		95.	☐	☐	☐	☐	☐
47.	☐	☐	☐	☐	☐		96.	☐	☐	☐	☐	☐
48.	☐	☐	☐	☐	☐		97.	☐	☐	☐	☐	☐
49.	☐	☐	☐	☐	☐							

EVALUATION OF TEXT AND TEST

Name: _____

Address: _____

City: _____ State: _____

Phone: (____) _____ ZIP: _____

Occupation: RN ☐   LPN ☐   EMT ☐
　　　　　　Paramedic ☐   Other _____

License # _____ State _____
Soc.Sec.# _____

How many hours did it take you to read the book and take the test: _____ hrs.

Did you find the material presented: *check all that apply*

☐ excellent　　☐ clear　　　　☐ well organized

☐ good　　　　☐ interesting　　☐ poorly organized

☐ fair　　　　 ☐ dull　　　　 ☐ too long

☐ poor　　　　☐ confusing　　☐ too short

Was the CEU test? *check all that apply*

☐ too hard　　☐ too long

☐ too easy　　☐ too short　　☐ about right

Thank you for your time. Any comments you would like to make are welcome. Any recommendation/suggestions for the 2nd edition would be appreciated.

12 Lead EKG STAT
A Light-Hearted Approach

An engaging *EKG FAIRYTALE* combined with
CARDIAC CARTOONS
totally destroy the intimidation and boredom
that usually accompany learning 12 lead EKGs

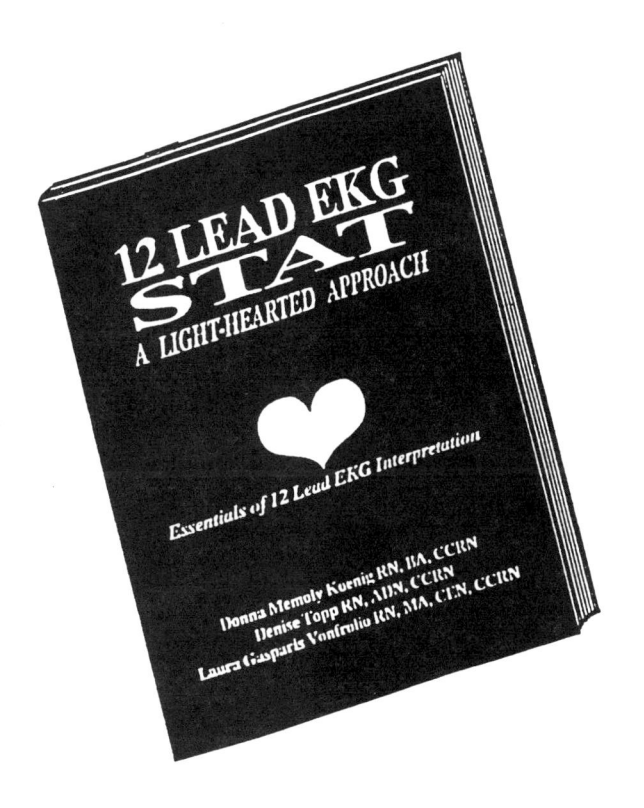

Have fun while you read this book!
Learn to interpret 12 lead EKGs in a systematic way.
Enjoy great illustrations
Earn CEUs upon completion of a post-test.

SEE ORDER FORM ON THE BACK OF THIS PAGE.

ORDER FORM
12 LEAD EKG STAT!
A LIGHT-HEARTED APPROACH

Make check or MO payable to: CEU ACCESS and mail to BOOKMASTERS 1444 US Route 42, RD. 11, Mansfield, OH 44903 or Call 1-800-247-6553 or Fax 1-419-281-6883.

I would like to order _____ copy(ies)
@ $19.95 each for $ _____

                Add postage & handling   3.00

                             Total $ _____

Please charge my Visa ☐   MC ☐ # _____ Exp. Date _____

Payment MUST accompany order . . . Thank You!

Name: _____

Address: _____

_____ Telephone _____

12 Lead EKG STAT
A Light-Hearted Approach

An engaging *EKG FAIRYTALE* combined with
CARDIAC CARTOONS
totally destroy the intimidation and boredom
that usually accompany learning 12 lead EKGs

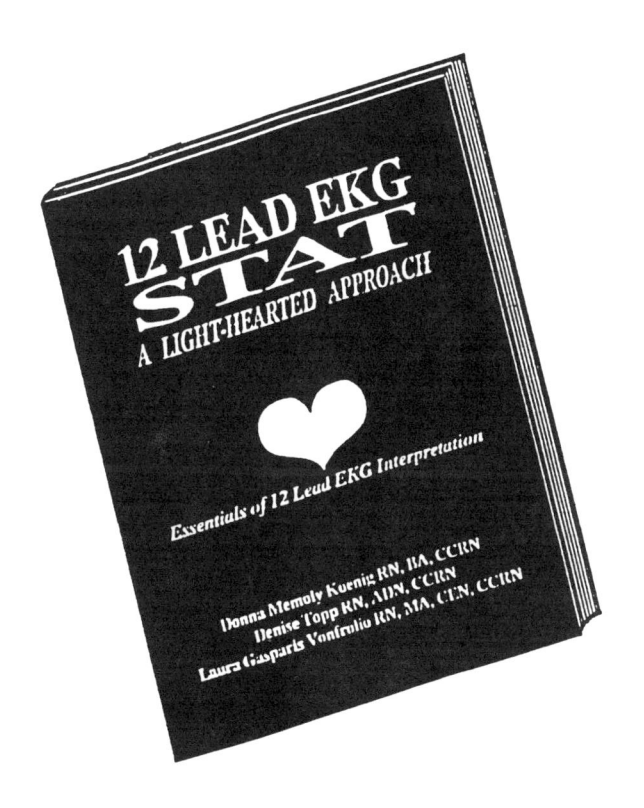

Have fun while you read this book!
Learn to interpret 12 lead EKGs in a systematic way.
Enjoy great illustrations
Earn CEUs upon completion of a post-test.

SEE ORDER FORM ON THE BACK OF THIS PAGE.

ORDER FORM
12 LEAD EKG STAT!
A LIGHT-HEARTED APPROACH

Make check or MO payable to: CEU ACCESS and mail to
BOOKMASTERS 1444 US Route 42, RD. 11, Mansfield, OH 44903
or Call 1-800-247-6553 or Fax 1-419-281-6883.

I would like to order _____ copy(ies)
@ $19.95 each for $ _____

Add postage & handling   3.00

Total $ _____

Please charge my Visa ☐   MC ☐   # _____   Exp. Date _____

Payment MUST accompany order . . . Thank You!

Name: _____

Address: _____

_____ Telephone _____

REVOLUTION
THE JOURNAL OF NURSE EMPOWERMENT

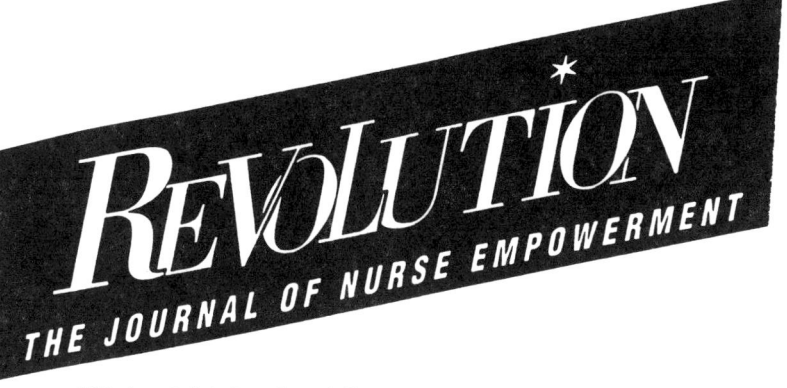

published quarterly by Laura Gasparis Vonfrolio & A. D. Von Publishers

If you feel the nursing profession is worth fighting for ...

Join The Revolution

A new journal that focuses on academic, clinical, personal, and political issues that affect Registered Nurses

We take on the "sacred cows"
- Academic programs that fail today's nursing needs
- The lack of law, business & ethics courses for nurses
- Sexism & sexual harrassment
- Feminism & nursing
- Legislative updates
- Financial advisement

Our goal is to help empower nurses to change the system:
- How to participate in activist issues
- How to affect legislation
- How to influence curricula
- How to transform hospital administrations
- How to handle intimidation and threats

Become part of a powerful force "the system" will have to reckon with...

Join the Revolution

Send $19.95 check or Money Order to:
A.D. Von Publishers, 56 Mc Arthur Avenue, Staten Island, New York 10312

OR CALL 1-800-331-6534 to charge on Visa / MC

NAME _____

ADDRESS _____

CITY _____ STATE _____ ZIP _____

SPECIALITY _____

NURSE ABUSE
IMPACT AND RESOLUTION

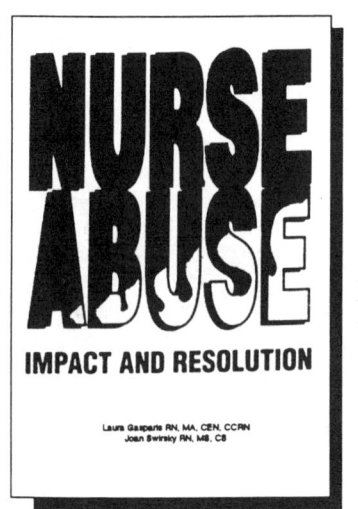

Laura Gasparis RN, MA, CEN, CCRN
Joan Swirsky RN, MS, CS

The book that's fast becoming the catalyst for meaningful changes in nursing

$19.95

The pervasive abuse of nurses permeates a system which begins with their academic and clinical training and continues into all the settings in which nurses work.

Undervalued, stereotyped, treated with cavalier indifference, and crass condescension, nurses are beginning to shout, "I'm fed up and I'm not going to take it anymore." The nationwide nursing shortage is a clear indication that nurses need to come out of the proverbial closet.

Authored by staff nurses, nurse administrators, professors of nursing and nurse researchers. This book focuses on the frustrations, problems and barriers confronting nurses, as well as offering solutions.

"NURSE ABUSE" is fast becoming the catalyst helping the noble art and science of nursing gain its rightful and respected place in the health care system.

ORDER TODAY
REMEMBER YOUR NURSE FRIENDS, MAKES A GREAT GIFT
Send check or Money Order to:
Power Publications, 56 Mc Arthur Avenue, Staten Island, New York 10312

NAME _____

ADDRESS _____

CITY _____ STATE _____ ZIP _____

SPECIALITY _____

Laura Gasparis Vonfrolio RN, MA, CEN, CCRN

CEN or CCRN REVIEW ON TAPE
MAKES CRAMMING EASY
Study the material over & over, anytime, anyplace

CCRN Revised for the 1992 exam

Recorded at an intensive one day seminar.

These tapes offer many tips on the style and content you can expect on the test.

Not a boring recitation of facts that you'll find offered by many others.

Laura's style is both entertaining and educational making the information more interesting and easier to remember..

CEN Review designed to improve your performance on the exam

A complete review of the exam for content and style with many valuable tips that will help you pass.

Presented in Laura's unique style that makes even the most difficult information easy to remember.

Edited from one of Laura's a one day, intensive, fast paced seminars.

IMPROVE YOUR PERFORMANCE
- PASS THE EXAM

NAME _____

ADDRESS _____

STATE _____ ZIP _____

☐ CCRN REVIEW TAPES – $49.95   ☐ CEN REVIEW TAPES – $49.95 $ _____

Sales Tax, (NY Residents Only) $ _____

Shipping & Handling $ 3.50

TOTAL $ _____

Make check payable to: Education Enterprises Send to 56 McArthur Avenue, Staten Island, NY 10312

PINNING JELLO TO A WALL

Leadership . . .
Empowerment . . .
Nurse Abuse . . .
Shared Governance . . .
What About Nursing?

Bob Hess will address these issues with your professional group or organization as a keynote speaker or inhouse consultant

Robert Hess, MSN, RN, CCRN, CNAA is an acclaimed international speaker and an award-winning writer, co-author of **Nurse Abuse: Impact and Resolution,** creator of the Pat Iyer tape on **Shared Governance,** and an editorial board member of **Revolution: The Journal of Nurse Empowerment.** Bob is a bedside nurse with over ten years' experience in nursing administration, and adjunct nursing faculty.

Contact:
Professional Care
Suite 400
10 Evergreen Drive
Voorhees, NJ 08043
(609) 424-4270

AUDIOTAPES AVAILABLE
from
PATRICIA IYER ASSOCIATES

Order today! Earn contact hours!

☐ **Liability Issues for Emergency Department Nurses**
This valuable tape will reduce your risk of being sued by helping you identify potential legal situations.
1.5 hrs (2 contact hrs) $16.95

☐ **Legal Aspects of Charting**
This best selling tape provides 20 guidelines for clear charting. It will update your knowledge of legal aspects of documentation. Nursing case law examples will help you apply the concepts presented.
1.5 hrs (2 contact hrs) $16.95

☐ **Team Building**
How do you create a more, cohesive team of nurses? You'll learn why team building is essential for improved care.
1 hr (1.5 contact hrs) $12.95

☐ **Become A Published Author**
Enhance your professional expertise through publishing. This tape provides tips for making your writing project a success. Learn how to develop an idea, organize a topic, prepare a manuscript and negotiate a book contract.
1 hr (1.5 contact hrs) $12.95

☐ **Handle The Angry Complainer**
How many times have you been confronted by an angry patient, family or doctor? This tape will increase your ability to obtain and act on complaints without becoming defensive.
1 hr (1.5 contact hrs) 12.95

☐ **Stress Management**
Are you stressed? You'll learn to recognize your own reactions to stress and those of other nurses when you listen to this humorous treatment of stress management. This tape is filled with practical suggestions for reducing your stress level.
1 hr (1.5 contact hrs) $12.95

☐ **Shared Governance**
Learn why shared governance is the hottest new management approach. This tape describes the advantages of this model and provides a practical method for selecting and implementing a shared governance model.
75 mins (2 contact hrs) $16.95

☐ **Implementing Nursing Quality Assurance Programs**
Learn more about unit-based nursing QA programs by listening to this experienced Nursing Quality Assurance Coordinator. The strategies in this tape will help you motivate and educate staff nurses.
1 hr (1.5 contact hrs) $12.95

☐ **Through The Eyes of The Law: Legal Aspects of Nursing Practice**
By listening to this live program, you'll be able to better identify liability issues specific to your clinical setting and take action to reduce your risk of being sued for malpractice. You'll learn important guidelines for documentation that will improve your charting. If you ever end up in a lawsuit, you'll be able to use techniques to comfortably answer questions in a deposition or trial.
4.5 hrs (6 contact hrs) $49.95

☐ **Nursing QA: The 10 Step Model**
You'll be able to explain the Joint Commission's Ten Step QA model and develop indicators to measure the important aspects of care in your setting.
1 hour (1.5 contact hrs) $12.95

☐ **Bioethics for Nurses**
Are you comfortable with resolving ethical issues? This often difficult and complex area is clearly explained by this tape.
1 hr (1.5 contact hrs) $12.95

☐☐☐☐☐☐☐☐☐☐☐☐☐

Patricia Iyer Associates is an approved provider of continuing education through NJSNA (#35-11-92) which is accredited by the American Nurses Association, and by the California Board of Registered Nursing (CEP 10146)

We have other tapes. Call or write for a complete listing!

ORDERING INFORMATION: Check the cassettes you want. Make check payable to Patricia Iyer Associates. Fill in name and address below and mail to Patricia Iyer Associates, 55 Britton Rd, Stockton, NJ 08559. **To earn contact hours add $10 to the price of each tape.** Questions? Call 908-788-8227 or fax to 908-806-4511.

Order Amount **Shipping Charges** Up to $16.95 $1.50 $17 - $35 $4.00 Over $35 $7.00 **Method of Payment:** ☐ Check ☐ Credit Card	Amt of Order: $ _____ Shipping Chg: $ _____ Contact Hours - ($10/tape): $ _____ TOTAL: $ _____

NAME:
ADDRESS:
CITY: STATE: ZIP:
DAY PHONE: (   )

CARD #:   EXPIRATION:
CARD HOLDER SIGNATURE:

TechniCardia®

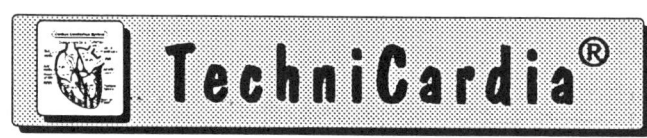

ARRHYTHMIA TUTORIAL SOFTWARE AND REFERENCE LIBRARY
The most comprehensive overview of cardiac arrhythmias currently available

Computer Assisted Instruction

Approved for 34 Contact Hours!

(CATEGORY A)

- No Computer Experience is Necessary
- AACN Approved for 3.4 CEUs - Category A
- Home Study Course Available - Includes Textbook
- Records and Tracks Test Scores
- FREE Updates and Technical Support

FREE TEN DAY EVALUATION*

-- ✂

☐ Yes! Please send TechniCardia Education package for free 10 day evaluation (*Institutions only please).

☐ Yes! Please send me the TechniCardia® Home Study Course IBM PC* version for use on my personal computer at $129.00 (DOS 2.0, EGA/VGA Monitor).

☐ Yes! Please send me the 12 LEAD EKG STAT! Software at $39.95 (See other side for more details!).

☐ My check is enclosed   Charge to my VISA or MasterCard

☐ Card #:_____   Exp.:_____

☐ Signature :_____   Date :_____

Please Print

Name:_____ Daytime Tel #: (   )_____
Address:_____
City:_____ State:_____ Zip:_____
Employed by:_____

Offer only good in the U.S. Prices outside the U.S. are slightly higher. All prices are subject to change without notice.

Shipment to PO Boxes must be prepaid. © Copyright 1991-92 GS Microsystems. All Rights Reserved.

AVAILABLE DECEMBER 1992

THE SOFTWARE VERSION

of this book!

12 LEAD EKG STAT
A LIGHTHEARTED APPROACH
The Essentials of 12 Lead EKG Interpretation

- No Computer Experience is Necessary to Use the Software
- Learn to Interpret 12 Lead EKG in a Systematic Way
- Great Graphics, Illustrations, Colors, Animation and Fun
- **SPECIAL INTRODUCTORY PRICE: ONLY $39.95**

Everything you always wanted to know about 12 Lead EKG's...but were too busy to ask! Now, it even runs on your computer!

POSTAGE

GS Microsystems

872 Hinckley Road
BURLINGAME CA 94010